The Loss of Self: Self-Writing as a Tool in Borderline Psychoanalysis

Jean-François Chiantaretto

Translated by Agnès Jacob

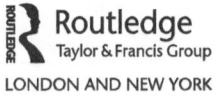

Routledge
Taylor & Francis Group

LONDON AND NEW YORK

Designed cover image: Georges Gaillard, Éphémères, 2017

First published in English 2025
by Routledge
4 Park Square, Milton Park, Abingdon, Oxon OX14 4RN

and by Routledge
605 Third Avenue, New York, NY 10158

Routledge is an imprint of the Taylor & Francis Group, an informa business

Published in French by SPF-CP/éditions Campagne Première as La
Perte de soi, 2020

British Library Cataloguing-in-Publication Data
A catalogue record for this book is available from the British Library

ISBN: 9781032893853 (hbk)
ISBN: 9781032893846 (pbk)
ISBN: 9781003542483 (ebk)

DOI: 10.4324/9781003542483

Typeset in Times New Roman
by codeMantra

The Loss of Self: Self-Writing as a Tool in Borderline Psychoanalysis

The Loss of Self considers distinctions and connections between the writing of survival and survival as a mode of being and thinking encountered in analytic work with borderline patients.

Jean-François Chiantaretto draws a parallel between Freud's use of writing in constructing the psychoanalytic edifice and the way each analyst may turn to writing when reflecting on a patient's analysis. With close reference to the writings of Imre Kertész, the book brings a unique perspective to the literary and historical concept of survival.

The Loss of Self will be of interest to psychoanalysts in practice and in training.

Jean-François Chiantaretto is a Paris-based psychoanalyst and professor emeritus of clinical psychopathology at Sorbonne Paris North University. Trained in philosophy and clinical psychology, he is a member and scientific secretary of the Quatrième Groupe.

To Catherine

Contents

Acknowledgements   *ix*
Foreword   *xi*
Prologue: Back and Forth Between Treatment and Writing   *xiii*

PART 1
The Beginnings   1

1 Unease about Origins, Unease at the Origins   3

2 The Original, the Originary   9

PART 2
Renewing Psychoanalysis   25

3 The Ferenczian Renewal   26

4 Beginning, Starting Over   40

5 Welcoming the Unwelcome Child   50

PART 3
Writing at the Borderline   61

6 Survival in Words   63

7 *Writing for…*   74

8 *Writing against…*   80

PART 4
Borderline Existence   87

  9 Disappearance *or* Loss   89

 10 From Culture to Treatment: Malaise in Transparency   98

     Epilogue: The Analyst's Transference, Transferential Writing   109
     Addendum: The Self in Question   113
     Index   123

Acknowledgements

Certain psychoanalytic encounters exerted their influence, in one way or another, on the conception and writing of this book: encounters with Jean-Luc Donnet, Fernando Geberovich, Suzanne Molnard, and Jean-Claude Rolland.

A "psychoanalytic encounter": meeting an analyst who helps one to find his own manner of being an analyst in the session, to write afterwards—staying or not staying faithful to the session—and to find alone, in the midst of the others, his own way of being.

I would also like to acknowledge Nathalie Zaltzman and Pierre Fédida, encountered too early and only from a distance; they were decisive intellectual interlocutors during the writing of *The Loss of Self*.

I am grateful to Janine Altounian and Catherine Matha, who were kind enough to read the manuscript, and made valuable remarks well beyond formal corrections.

My thanks also go to my colleagues and friends in the group "*Littérature personnelle et psychanalytique*" (1992–2018) who have accompanied me since the group was created: Janine Altounian, Nicole Beauchamp, Anne Clancier (now deceased), Mireille Fognini, Antonia Fonyi, Ghyslain Levy, Josette Pacaly, Jacqueline Rousseau-Dujardin, Arnaud Tellier—with a special thought for Jacqueline, who left us not long ago.

Foreword

I have long been interested in self-writing, initially as a reader and later as a reader and psychoanalyst. This interest, unexamined at first, has no doubt contributed greatly to creating a distance between myself and philosophy, particularly the Frankfurt School of Critical Theory. Given that my training was in philosophy, I had sought a middle road in aesthetics and literature, through the Brechtian concept of "intervening thought." The idea of writing as a thinking process, not reducible to the transcription of thoughts, was already present, but it was only when I encountered Freud, as a clinical psychologist and later as an analyst, that I started to examine more closely the question of self-presentation in writing.

But more than seeing self-presentation as an autobiographical model, it was when I realised the extent to which Freud relied on writing to create psychoanalysis that I was able to formulate clearly my notion of self-writing, in 1995. Several more years were needed before I understood fully the clinical foundation of Freud's recourse to writing:[1] a dialogue with himself, making the other witness to thinking in progress.

Self-presentation as found in self-writing (autobiography, diary, self-fiction, essay …) is necessarily a blend. It is founded on a narcissistic investment of words which supposedly convey to someone (the reader) how someone else (the author) sees himself. By means of this artifice, the self-presentation stages the passage[2]—with its impediments—from a subject's internal monologue, practically a soliloquy, to an internal dialogue requiring listening (reading) by another. Indeed, in my view, in this type of text, self-presentation is to be considered a certified authentic presentation of an internal dialogue, summoning the intrapsychic figure of a witness: the "internal witness," according to a hypothesis I formulated in 1999 based on *The Diary* of Anne Frank.

This proposition implies seeing internal dialogue as emerging at the intersection of writing and clinical work, where it becomes the scene of survival while posing a challenge. Since as far back as 2005 (if not earlier), the focus of my work has gone back and forth between writing by survivors (Primo Levi and Imre Kertész) and survival as a mode of being and thinking in borderline pathologies.

Consenting to the risk of the loss of self in the relation with the other proves to be desirable for everyone. Undefined loss of self is the reverse of undefined construction of self, involving more or less fortunate encounters with one's internal otherness and the otherness of others—in the plurality of the elements composing human beings: identificatory and relational, narcissistic and sexual. To live is to lose, until death and beyond death's intervention. Every person *owes it to himself* to consent to dying, in the process of living; to consent to the loss of self in the choice of possibilities and in the possible loss of another, which likely announces the loss of narcissistic investments associated with every relationship.

However, this internal loss is of an entirely different nature in borderline psychopathologies with melancholic or melancholiform aspects: here, there is loss of self in the other who has lost himself. Or, in more specifically psychoanalytic terms, the incorporation by the *infans* of the disappearance of the other essential to himself, if we follow the path laid out by Ferenczi. How can one survive this initial loss of self? This is the question inherent in "borderline existence," a question discussed throughout this book.

When psychoanalysis came into being, there was, of course, Freud and his initial transference onto writing. But there was also the first "new start" distinct from all the new beginnings that followed, up to the present day: the original/originary dialogue between Freud and Ferenczi. It was an impossible but productive dialogue, destructive and creative, into which every psychoanalyst must enter the concrete reality of his clinical practice, whether he wants to or not, and whether he writes or not.

I believe that giving this dialogue the attention it deserves allowed me to reexamine clinical work with borderline states. The specific difficulties of this psychoanalytic work enabled me to clarify the central role of "internal dialogue" in the psychic functioning of the analyst, in the session and—afterwards and differently—through writing *based on* the session.

I might also have gained an additional benefit: a certain *detachment* in regard to the *subject* of self-writing and the passion-fraught misunderstandings occasioned by the word "self," even setting aside its multiple usage. This could explain the choice of the book's title.

Notes

1 Beyond the diversity of its forms.
2 With or without the author's awareness, to an indefinite extent and in an infinitely variable manner depending on the text, even in the case of texts written by the same author.

Prologue

Back and Forth Between Treatment and Writing[1]

In Imre Kertész's writing, self-presentation institutes absence *as* a loss: the texts exhibit his self-effacement. But self-effacement transformed into a scene of writing becomes a saving action. When a witness depicts in writing an inhibition to be, he creates the possibility of being seen and heard. To tell someone, to describe the events in order to survive loss and render absence bearable, is also—albeit very differently—what characterises self-presentation in Pierre Pachet's *Autobiographie de mon père* (*My Father's Autobiography*). This book is written specifically *for* his dead father, to draw him out, *post mortem*, of the disappearance to himself he experienced while alive as a result of illness. This disappearance had the effect of amplifying the traumatic effacement caused by the Holocaust.

Literature helps the psychoanalyst transform what escapes him into the motif and material of his thinking, during and after the session. For the past ten years, the constant rereading of Kertész's work has played a decisive role[2] in helping me reflect on the central subject of this book: the melancholic dimension seen in borderline patients—the loss of self in the other, the investment of the self, perceived as *disappearing* in the other's thought.

The melancholic backdrop of transference, combined with the absence of the transferential object, brought about by the analyst, plays a very particular role for borderline patients. They literally cast doubt on the "depressive capacity" of the analytic situation in which "to hear is the equivalent of a loss," bringing into question the "depressivity of fantasy."[3]

How can the analyst maintain associations and representations with these patients, who impose on themselves and on him the melancholic resonance of disappearance, to counter the depressivity of absence? How can the analyst separate from his thoughts, which are set apart while bringing them together, how can he reflect on the activation of the anguish of loss brought about by absence, when the patient's need for self-effacement in the other solicits him? For, by denying the internal alterity of the other (the analyst), the patient aims at killing himself in the other, at proving that he is not there—an action that paradoxically dispenses him from having to make himself disappear, from killing himself. This allows the patient to survive the threat of annihilation existing at the earliest period of the unwelcome infant's history, to use Ferenczi's terms. Keeping in mind that the threat was inscribed in the infant's psyche in the extreme form of an internal injunction, pronounced by no one!

In this clinical context, how is it possible to take the risk of abstaining from transferential role attribution in interpretation? How can the analyst invest the patient's passage from the unthinkable pain of being to the unbearable suffering of living, while assuming the danger of the (suicidal) temptation of becoming the willing protagonist of his own disappearance? This question, difficult to conceive in the session, becomes clear when the analyst looks at the sessions from the outside, specifically through the act of writing; it can then become the source of torment that obliterates words, preventing writing and even erasing it ...

To tell someone, to speak for someone, sometimes to tell in order to live an unliveable absence punctured by loss ... This is, generally speaking, the hope of every analysand, admitted or denied, and in the best case ultimately deceived, through the capacity for absence in reaction to the analyst's psychic presence to himself—on the Winnicottian model of the mother who can be alone in the presence of her child, who, as a result, can discover his ability to play alone in her presence: to be alone.[4]

To speak for someone, to tell someone, to shape absence into a text, might have resembled what Freud expected, and certainly what Ferenczi expected when they addressed themselves to each other, prompting reciprocal reflection regarded as an expectation. Awareness of this originary reciprocity in psychoanalysis has, in any case, confirmed my view of the analyst's *internal dialogue* in the session. Internal dialogue, that is, how the analyst speaks to himself in the session, how this internal dialogue in context reflects the modalities through which he puts it into words, and how it is reflected in the interpretations he offers to the patient.

The unspeakable can be seen as signalling the urgency of a transfer of self-destructiveness, an initial appeal demanding the immediate disposition to receive, the threat to life activated by the patient's request, a threat revealing the melancholic depths of his psyche. In transference, in order to make possible the unprecedented confrontation requested by the patient, the analyst is forced to withstand alone the attack of his thinking process, and to survive it by becoming conscious of the work of aggressivity in himself. He must survive *then and there*, in that particular confrontation, and above all not only elsewhere, with other patients or in his personal life; he must survive *this*, the experience of the unspeakable as a sign of the unliveable. The request of the borderline patient implies action. It is expressed in a transferential induction, which takes the form of an insurmountable tension felt by the analyst, to be borne as it is: the tension between making or not making a libidinal investment in the patient as a new source of affects and thoughts. Indeed, the borderline sphere prompts the analyst to write as forcefully as it stops him from writing. The only desirable outcome would be either to succeed in inscribing negatively through the process of writing the effacement induced by the patient—to (partially) invest writing as a place of survival—or to find an equivalent for putting effacement in writing by creating thirdness in supervision or through the use of any other inter-analytic device.

In this context, we are no longer dealing with neurotic inhibition of thought—not unrelated to the nature of the thinking process itself. To think, or more specifically to think creatively, to invest thinking as a creative experience, means to think in the very place where thought eludes us and renders us absent to ourselves; that is, to assert the primacy of the symbolisation of absence over the possibility of disappearance, to risk producing anxiety instead of bearing the anguish of loss. This is the difference between the thought of murder characteristic of the oedipal/neurotic sphere, and the murder of thought, characterising what Paul-Claude Recamier, following in Ferenczi's footsteps, calls incestuality, a central element in borderline pathologies and psychoses.

Every analysis is expected to bring the analyst face to face with anxiety sooner or later, to a greater or lesser extent. This anxiety is related to the mutual identifications inherent to transference: how to avoid being lost in the patient's identifications, and in identifications to the patient? The analyst's thought process and, as a last resort, recourse to his countertransferential affects, is what makes it possible to render this reciprocity creative by materialising the dissymmetry of places and the separation of psychic spaces. In other words, it is the analyst's thought process that establishes the differentiation from the places assigned in and by transference, which ultimately means the differentiation between the patient *and* himself. Someone is listening, someone in the analyst and beyond him is listening to both the patient and the analyst. I have named this thought process "potential writing":[5] work done from a perspective on the session stemming from the session, a beyond-the-session in the session, like the anticipation of writing to come. This accomplishes the inscription of the analyst's acknowledged solitude: he is alone with the patient, alone in the presence/absence of the *symbolic* analytic community, given form by the internal dialogue with his own transferential figures.

This point of view enables the analyst to forgo embodying the interlocutor the patient is asking for, while acquiescing to his request by acting as a witness in transference. Transference determines and is determined by the analyst's internal dialogue, defined as an internal experience equivalent to the self-observation of theorisation in progress, whose stages are undone so that this undoing/retraction of the previously thought can let an unprecedented interpretation emerge.[6] Interpretation is inseparable from self-interpretation, but goes beyond it, in principle. This is only true if the analyst pursues an internal dialogue—in fact, it is what allows him to have this dialogue, to see himself and experience himself in the immediacy of the session. This is how his thought process provides the analyst with a place for working through counter-transferential affects and metabolising the anxiety inherent to the analytic situation—a place without which interpretive activity could not be translated into interpretation.

In Fédida's theoretical perspective which posits a "site of the stranger,"[7] this anxiety can be connected to the encounter with the stranger, which activates the many facets of *strangeness*, referring back to endless combinations of the strange and the stranger: the stranger in oneself and in the other, as well as strangeness to oneself, in both. The analytic process involves the mobilisation of the analyst's and analysand's internal alterity: four people take part in the analysis, producing an indefinite number of *identificatory combinations*, not intended, strictly speaking, to acquire the consistency of a relationship or an encounter.

The analysis takes place in an in-between space of shared intimacy, a space not belonging to one or the other, nor to both, but involving both, albeit unequally, since this in-between space is asymmetrically guaranteed by the analyst's thought process. The analyst's anguish is structural and necessary, for it is connected with "a kind of mourning for oneself that requires another presence,"[8] which the analyst ensures for the patient and for himself.

If we conclude that the site of the stranger is language, I would say that it is, even more specifically, the analyst's internal dialogue. In the session, this dialogue materialises his thought process in words, calling forth the patient's renewed or unprecedented internal experience of his alterity. The analyst's internal dialogue in the session materialises his thought process in an internal dialogue with others, sparked by the patient's numerous transferential figures, intersecting with the numerous figures involved in his own transference, figures associated with his past experience as an analysand, with his life experience and with his reflection in general. This dialogue is the space and the instrument of an alternation through the alterity of words and in the words: it sets in motion the intimate contact between words, the feeling of being alive, through the forfeiting of words as well as through surrendering to words, indissociably in oneself and between oneself and the other.

This anxiety-filled encounter with the stranger is what is forfeited with borderline patients, desperately true to themselves through a hatred desperately transferred *into* the other, since it cannot be addressed directly. For those who survived an early rupturing of the environment—a hole in the psychic presence of the primordial (first) other—survival will *forever* be dependent on the other's ability to survive the hate they transfer into him. Forced to live in hate, the other is expected to protect the borderline subject from the threat of melancholia associated with the incorporation of self-denial inflicted on oneself. My view of the melancholic aspect of borderline psychopathology falls within the Ferenczian perspective of narcissistic self-splitting.[9]

Here, incorporation stems from the narcissistic injury in the environment, at the initial time of the *Hilflösigkeit*, from the danger felt then of disappearing in the disappearance of the other to himself—an other on whom the infant depended for his very life. The formulation of this hypothesis was based on François Perrier's idea of a "denial of oneself imposed by oneself,"[10] although his concept concerned the specific problem of alcoholism and addictions in general. The hypothesis presented in my book is based on the idea of a link characterised by the inaugural incorporation by the *infans* of the disappearance of the other to himself, when "the other" is the primordial or first other, relative to the infant's state of vital dependence, or, to use a term closer to Freud's (*Hilflösigkeit*), the infant's helplessness, in Laplanche's terminology. This incorporation will establish the type of relation to the other characteristics of borderline structure in adulthood.

The hatred of the borderline subject is there to force the other into effacement *and* to force him to fight against it, that is, to force him to prove his non-disappearance twice over. This prevents the subject from being overwhelmed by his own disappearance into the other, as was his experience at a very early stage, and as he tries to repeat it—in an act of narcissistic *self-splitting*, a division of the being between the hope of making this disappearance thinkable by the other, and the expectation that the other will give him sufficient confirmation of guilt, for him to attach his self-destructiveness to it and continue to survive in hate. And when the other is the analyst, his potential writing in the session creates a space that can take in the survivor of the murder committed against himself, of the deadly splitting of the ego. Potential writing is the *transcription* by the analyst, in response to the patient's transference, of the internal dialogue bringing together the very mixed internal cohort of his transferential figures and the symbolic analytic community.

There will be someone to carry out self-effacement, and someone to fight against it. But the fight against effacement must never be won definitively. *Never*: not before the patient is able to let go of the anguish of loss—as the sign of a disappearance announced by the infant's experience of the disappearance of his primordial other—in favour of the anguish brought by the stranger, or, to be more exact, before he is able to tolerate the advent of the second type of anguish.

* * *

In this particular clinical context, taking notes after the session allows the analyst to assert to himself that he is offering enough resistance to effacement, but not too much. The notes are intended only to keep a trace of what he experiences in the session, through what he says to himself—which helps him to bear having to face, in the next session, the patient's attempts at bringing about effacement. But the silent violence of transferential attributions makes it difficult to establish the right balance with certainty.

Resistance to note-taking, leading to almost no notes at all, could be considered, in the most difficult cases, a forced defensive solution as much as a necessary compromise, at least for a time. It would maintain the possibility of writing as a thinking process, creating absence instead of a void, and introducing the possibility of effacement rather than disappearance. I shall describe a specific instance that illustrates well the type of difficulty encountered with such patients: a case where, after being governed by an uncontrollable prohibition to take notes, I felt just as strongly that I had to write. Specifically, I felt forced to look, by writing, for confirmation that my thinking process not only survived, but had remained lively, at least relatively speaking. And not merely in note-taking, but in published work. In other words, the internal constraint led to undertaking to write as a countertransferential act.

The patient in question[11] caused me such concern and worry that I decided to go back to working under supervision. This patient embodied quite dramatically the pain of being attached to the self-destructiveness typical of borderline functioning—which Schreber aptly called "soul murder"—that is, the carrying out against oneself a psychic murder prompted by the other: the reception of the deadly hatred of the other for himself, *re-addressed* to oneself. How can absence be introduced in such a configuration?

With this patient, recourse to writing became necessary in order to overcome elsewhere the threat of disappearance inscribed in the sessions. This threat made the effacement demanded by the transference impossible to bear, because it attacked too violently the analyst's ability to *detach* from the object of transference, to create absence.

To be more precise, the analyst turned to writing to restore the inner scene of internal dialogue. This required writing to testify to this scene as possibly including an experience of creativity in conceiving of destructivity, following the example of the internal dialogue in Freud's work *and* between Freud and Ferenczi. No doubt, this witnessing needed to be foreseen, and even authorised in the space of thirdness provided by the supervision. But by placing absence elsewhere, the analyst's writing took the risk of strengthening the tendency to suicidal action: the risk that the search for disappearance could lead to a successful suicide attempt.

This caused me to re-examine Freud's notion of the work of melancholia, elevated to the status of a concept by Benno Rosenberg,[12] in the form of a distinction between the relinquishing of self and detachment from oneself. The latter is said to define the melancholic aspect of the borderline sphere, in a particular narcissistic investment of the object. The "borderline subject" is condemned never to find himself in the object, and therefore to lose himself in the self-hatred discharged into the other. By contrast, detachment from oneself is the result of the work enabling passage from the indissoluble attachment of self and the other, to "detachability," as Rosenberg called it. In a borderline context, the work of melancholia seems related to self-effacement aimed at fighting against disappearance, against the temptation of making oneself disappear, against the coercion of being the actor of one's own disappearance in order to rid oneself of the incorporation of one who vanished, to discard the disappearance that another inflicted on himself. But the work of melancholia, seen as the *ultimate fight* against the threat of melancholia, can only be done by the patient when facilitated by the analyst. This is where the difficulty lies, since the analyst has to let the poison of effacement act upon him and against him, until he is filled with the void which *undoes* the other, silently and invisibly, at the sources of the possible suicidal action of the patient—until he is filled with it *and* transforms it into anguish.

Between the threat of suicidal action on the part of a borderline patient wishing to make himself disappear instead of *being made to disappear*, and the fear of seeing himself disappear in the transference, which activates self-effacement in the analyst, there is a big difference. The patient must at all cost feel excluded from this sphere of difference: the shared sphere of thought with its libidinal sources. The analyst is able to benefit from allied individuals present in him, starting with colleagues he consults. As a result, consent to self-effacement of thought at its intimate roots—partial yet likely to attack the analyst's deepest being—could be liveable: possible to delimit in oneself and thus potentially representable, at least laterally, on the side.

In these cases, how can the analyst make a place in himself, *for the sake of the patient*, for the one who disappeared and who threatens him with disappearance in the transference? How can he do this without being overly absent, or effacing himself too much, when his own propensity to effacement is so insistently solicited by the patient? In other words, how can the analyst create an absence in himself *for the patient*? In the situation to which I refer here, the outcome was an act of writing, following the inhibition of writing as a thinking process—the hindrance of notes as a materialisation of the self-effacement making it possible to delimit and to limit effacement.

* * *

In psychoanalysis, hate and love, commonly called transference hate and love, best reveal their enigmatic nature when the analyst starts to write, if he is willing to see, in the words he writes, evidence of the feelings that underlie his internal dialogue in the session. The analyst's internal dialogue puts into words a number of ever-renewed polarities, a space stretching between two poles: love and hate, need and desire, sending out and taking in, being active or passive, difference and similarity, separation and reception … Speech in listening and listening to speech. These different modalities are no doubt more easily recognisable in less complex clinical situations than the one described here.

The analyst's two-in-one internal dialogue is part of the setting in place of the in-between[13] created by the *one for two* of the (counter)transferential offer that responds in advance to a transferential request—a "one for two" to which the analyst's writing testifies, when he has the courage to write, that is, when he risks testifying to the *half-repression* at work in his internal dialogue in the session; when he does so consenting to testify neither *about* nor *for* the analysand, without taking possession of the space of the analysis, but rather to give his version of the between-the-two of transference and counter-transference, thus leaving room for a different potential version, that of the patient.

Thus, the analyst testifies in and through *after-writing*—that is, from an elsewhere he alone articulates—to the thirdness at work in his internal dialogue in the session. By doing this, he renders readable something of the intractably enigmatic nature of the functioning of each protagonist, and of their relation. Here, the *one for two* holds a place exactly opposite to the *one in two* of non-separation, of the imaginary completeness that the actions of borderline patients strive to maintain, since in their case fear of loss takes precedence over castration anxiety. In more general terms, beyond the specific requirements of the borderline sphere, the aim of writing based on the session is to reveal the work of internal dialogue through a clinical presentation that consents to put in writing the role played by desire in the elaboration of counter-transference. This work uncovers the transference underlying it: the analyst's transference not only as a response to the patient's transference, but as an offer of transference preceding and influencing that of the latter.

In an analysis, what is essential centres around the analysand's ability to *create*, on his own and in his relation with the analyst, between sessions, in his inner life and his relationships, what he *finds* with the analyst in the sessions—that is, the creative possibilities of the deferred response of the analyst to his own transferential request. This capacity to be alone in the absence or presence of the other proves to be more or less inadequate in borderline cases. Therefore, it has to be acquired by the patient; he must gradually learn to bear the in-between interval separating transference and counter-transference, to consent to participate in the latter *as well*, and to accept that he will be definitively influenced by the analyst's *internal* dialogue.

The analyst's internal dialogue influences his patients' experience of interiority—first the other's—as a distance between oneself and the other, as well as within oneself: between oneself and one's representation of self, by oneself and by the other. In the session, the analyst speaks to himself, he listens to his listening to the other; to do this, he needs an internal interlocutor: a figure made up of a thousand identificatory figures, which enlarges his interiority, going beyond it, in the words and through the two-in-one experience.

Going beyond: what the protagonists discover, together and separately, what brings them together and separates them. In more conventional terms, this *beyond* could be called thirdness or the third function of the setting, as it is guaranteed and supported by the analyst's internal dialogue—which materialises in the silent words of the latter the two-in-one of his internal space. This perspective should doubtless be applied to the reconsideration of numerous questions about counter-transference with which analysts are still struggling today, in controversies centring primarily on borderline situations.

For a long time, psychoanalysts have opposed too systematically Freud's idea of neutrality and the primacy of scientific imperatives, and Ferenczi's mutual analysis and the primacy of therapeutic requirements. But this framework is always needed when the analyst's mirror function and his empathic function have to be opposed, when, as I see it, clinical work with borderline patients makes it necessary to conceive of opposition in terms of polarity rather than exclusion. Sexual and narcissistic aspects in the analyst, invested in the investigation of the patient's psychic functioning—presuming that the latter proceeds to self-examination of his own psyche, always characterise analytic treatment. But in a borderline context, it becomes the central element of the process.

The analytic scene activates the analyst's and the analysand's internal alterity. Between them and in *each one* of them, the means and objective of the therapeutic work consist of making shared creativity possible. This creativity specific to the treatment produces thousands of points of intersection of their respective internal scenes, but it is the task of the analyst to facilitate for the analysand a better delimitation of his being and easier access to its depth: better presence to himself.

In the borderline sphere, this involves experiencing and attacking the resistance of the analyst's internal alterity—his ability to think of the survival and creative transformation of the self-destructive tendency of the other in oneself. It is on this condition that such patients can gain access to the denied or disavowed distress associated with incestual hate. This is what makes it possible to reawaken the secret link between infantile sexuality and the relational component of the being.

Notes

1 This prologue renews, in the perspective of the present book, certain propositions presented in Chiantaretto, J.-F., Martha, C., and Neau, F. (Eds.), *L'Écriture du psychoanalyste*, Hermann, 2018, pp. 59–73.

2 Including making me realise, recently, the intensity of the initial shock—forgotten since 1995—of discovering Pachet's text. I wrote an account of this in Chiantaretto, J.-F., *De l'acte autobiographique*, Champ Vallon, 1995. I will quote here, as a tribute and with gratitude, a passage that has stayed with me since: "What exactly did I lose? What was taken away from me? A taste for life drove me to look for it. I undertook this search using precisely what my father taught me: I turned to my 'inner life'. The instrument was there, it was what I inherited from my father … What my dead father had to say was asking to speak through me, like it had never spoken, beyond our joint force" (Pachet, P., *Autobiographie de mon père*, Belin, 1987, pp. 6–7).

3 Fedida, P. *Des bienfaits de la dépression: éloge de la psychothérapie*, Odile Jacob, 2001. See Chapter 3.

4 Winnicott, D. W., "The Capacity to Be Alone," *International Journal of Psycho-Analysis*, 39, 1958: 416–420.

5 See Chiantaretto, J.-F., "L'Écriture du psychoanalyste et la séance," in André, J. and Lasvergnas, I. (Eds.), *La Psychoanalyse à l'épreuve du malentendu*, PUF, 2006. Text of conference given in Montreal in 2002.

6 Piera Aulagnier's concept of "floating theorizing" is very valuable in this context. Much could also be said about Jean-Claude Rolland's concept of "internal dialogue." The term refers to a preconscious "agency needed to turn observation into theory," when the "internal dialogue" designates an internal experience as unavoidable. See Rolland, J.-C. (Ed.) "Un rêve de petit pan de mur jaune," in Gantheret, F. and Pontalis, J.-B. (Ed.), *Parler avec l'étranger*, Gallimard, 2003; Rolland, J.-C., "Observation clinique, construction théorique, pensée métapsychologique, trois étapes de la connaissance," *Libres cahiers pour la psychanalyse*, 9, 2004: pp. 87–108.

7 Fédida, P., *Le site de l'étranger* (The Site of the Stranger), Paris: PUF, 1995.

8 Fédida, P., *Le site de l'étranger* (The Site of the Stranger), Paris: PUF, 1995, p. 4.

9 See Ferenczi, S., "Confusion of the Tongues Between the Adult and the Child," *The International Journal of Psychoanalysis*, 30, 1949: 225–230.

10 Perrier, F., *La Chaussée d'Antin, Œuvre psychanalytique II*, Albin Michel, 2008, p. 503.

11 See the clinical situation *infra*: Welcoming the Unwelcome Child.

12 Rosenberg, B., *Massochisme mortifère et massochisme gardien de vie* (Deadly Masochism and Life-Preserving Masochism), Paris: PUF, 1991.

13 "What is analytic treatment if not … simply activating the in-between, between the analysandandhis analyst?" Jullien, F., *L'Écart et l'entre*, Galilée, 2012, pp. 65–66.

Part 1

The Beginnings

Chapter 1

Unease about Origins, Unease at the Origins

"What thou hast inherited from thy fathers, Acquire it to make it thine": this Freudian quote from Goethe's *Faust* has been cited so often among psychoanalysts that it has become very familiar. But we have yet to consider how strange this familiarity is, on many levels, and how clearly it testifies to our familiarity with the *Unheimlich* ...

* * *

This quote is generally used as a sign or a signal of complicity between psychoanalysts, as if it were a matter of asserting a shared Freudian identity. As if Goethe became the witness vouching for the analysts' capacity to inherit from Freud—a capacity always in danger of turning into an appropriation of Freud, in the worst sense of the word: reducing Freud to *our* Freud, that is, a proprietary meaning determined by the logic of affiliation and belonging. This, despite the fact that psychoanalysts are perfectly aware that they will never own Freud: the Freudian corpus, which reveals each text to be the work of a multiple Freud, shows from the start that it belongs to no one, not even to Freud. The relentless divisions of the analytic movement attest to this, and each patient reminds us of it in the strangeness of the transference. For Freud's invitation to think is simply inexhaustible, and each analysis is unprecedented and constitutes a renewed proposition to think.

But psychoanalysts can repress what they cannot ignore, and can even ignore it in their actions. They can repress the impossibility of appropriating Freud, through identification not so much with Freud but with his identifications—in this case with Goethe—as long as it's clear that this is to be considered an identification *through* Freud's identification with Goethe. Thus, Goethe is asked to be the witness who vouches for an identity or, to put it differently, to stand witness to a personal conviction regarding the unity and indivisible character of the psychoanalyst's ego, equated in the imagination with psychoanalysis. This postulates an inalienable *home*, *mine/ours* marked out and possessed once and for all: psychoanalysis considered one and indivisible.

Of course, repression can change into an act when the goal is to take possession of the Freudian heritage by excluding others—with the added advantage, therefore,

DOI: 10.4324/9781003542483-2

of bypassing a personal conquest, made with and despite one's own resistance to psychoanalysis. This leads to differentiation from others, to one's disqualification and possible exclusion, so that identifying the non-self will ensure the narcissistic coherence of the ego—in strange resonance again with the definition of the ego in *Beyond the Pleasure Principle*. The corollary to this will be the elimination of the Freudian common ground, and therefore the loss of its function as a third element.

Rather than taking ownership of Freud by making him inaccessible to other analysts, one should acquire him for oneself, personally. Freud cited Goethe in *An Outline of Psycho-Analysis*, begun just after he arrived in London, and left, as we know, unfinished. *An Outline* is Freud's testament in a manner of speaking, in which he bequeaths that to which his successors *must*, presumably, become heirs. This injunction to inherit issued by the superego is particularly noteworthy since the quote from Goethe appears in the last chapter, which discusses the superego, just before the last sentence where the superego is redefined as a psychic legacy, in a very particular manner:

> In the establishment of the super-ego we have before us, as it were, an example of the way in which the present is changed into the past ...[1]

"The present changed into the past": the concept deserves comment at least in regard to the theory of the superego. I shall examine it in light of Freud's notion of a legacy, not in terms of a psychoanalytic theory of inheritance, but in terms of psychoanalysis considered a legacy to acquire. My perspective will be double: on the one hand, the creative psychoanalytic cure, which Freud saw as an internal obligation to acquire the repressed, deposited in the self by others; on the other hand, the injunction addressed to psychoanalysts to acquire the Freudian corpus in order to inherit it. This reveals another aspect of the strange familiarity of the quote from Goethe. Freud does not cite Goethe's next sentence,[2] although it is essential to the question of heritage: "What you don't use is a dead weight, What's worthwhile is what you spontaneously create."[3]

Speaking of the creative process, we remember Freud's astonishing position in what I called his auto-biography in 1995,[4] the self-representation put forth in *The History of the Psychoanalytic Movement* and *The Origin and Development of Psychoanalysis*. These two versions of Freud's founding principles claim to constitute a text bringing together, and even to make coincide, the history of the birth of psychoanalysis, his own history as the first analyst, and his autobiography. Both essays present an account of the origins of psychoanalysis, where Freud puts in writing his phantasy of being the only witness to the conception of psychoanalysis.

Thus, putting the origins in writing literally creates a primal scene: all psychoanalysts are invited to witness the conception of psychoanalysis with Freud, through his testimony to the fact of his absence to himself in the creative act. The entire Freudian oeuvre invites analysts to recognise themselves in it as they undertake the process of becoming analysts—to recognise themselves in written texts which are themselves written in the first person. Becoming an analyst requires acquaintance with Freud's work. *As if it were a matter of repeating Freud's initial absence to himself*: an internal compulsion to repeat, while in a state of paradoxical expectation of a return of the repressed which would set in motion at long last a process of working through by means of identification with Freud, and by Freud himself. *As if* this work needed to be done for Freud as much as for oneself.

Of course, this transferential illusion hides and reveals, in its *exclusive* relation to Freud, the particularity of the analyst's transference to those who were his masters—a transference that remains ongoing and remains to be worked through in each patient's analysis.

In fact, the working through of this type of transference could be seen as personal raw material in the sublimation process underlying transference onto psychoanalysis. Still, illusion is what best illustrates the change of the present into the past in the testamentary definition of the superego given in *An Outline*, as we mentioned earlier.

When he gives the injunction to inherit, stemming from the superego, Freud seems to invite creative transference to his work, as an obligation for one who is an analyst. But the omission of Goethe's second sentence in the quote given by Freud is especially strange, given that the sentence concerns the birth of creativity. Undoubtedly, this omission reflects Freud's ambivalence, until the end, about a biographical approach to his work, as well as his desire to keep control of "the history of psychoanalysis." But another directly related question is that of his ambivalence towards his heirs, who might be tempted to create without him and without reference to him: to renew psychoanalysis without him, and even claim to reinvent it.

It is not likely that Freud's omission is related to his initial transference to writing and what this implies in terms of a fundamental relation of all analysts to writing, whether they happen to write or not. This transference has its source in Freud's envy of the writer, whom he considers able to imagine and describe repression without having to overcome it, contrary to the psychoanalyst and, above all, to the first theoretician of repression. From this point of view, each analyst inherits a personal relation to writing, that is, a specific experience of the intimacy of writing and of speech in psychoanalytic treatment—again—whether or not he writes. The essential thing is the status granted to this intimacy, which could be seen as the power to change loss into absence.[5]

Since psychoanalysts are inevitably faced with this intimacy, whether they know it or not, are they condemned to identification or counter-identification with Freud's envy of writers? The fact is that some analysts look for a personal way of writing based on what they experience in the analytic situation, which can take the form of writing aimed at clarifying certain aspects of the analytic process, or a form of writing unrelated to analytic treatment. In either case, a mode of self-representation is *explicitly* involved, regardless of the literary form, be it essay or novel, and including all the combinations of what I call self-writing—that is, different types of self-referential writing—and different forms of fiction.

The author who best represents this is Didier Anzieu, author of *Becket et le psy-chanalyste*, although a few more recent names could be mentioned.

* * *

Be that as it may, most psychoanalysts opt for one of three defensive positions[6] in regard to the fact that it was through transference to writing that Freud invented, indissociably, psychoanalysis and a personal manner of writing *I*.

The first option is to forgo writing emerging from the sessions, on the grounds that writing cannot be faithful to speech exchanged in the course of the treatment, which can only be transmitted and revealed, other than in the analysand's direct experience, within an intra-analytic or supervisory structure related to analytic training. The second option consists of renouncing the search for a personal manner of writing "I," choosing an identity-conferring form of belonging rather than an identificatory form, either by writing *like* someone—Lacan, Winnicott, etc.—or by attempting to reduce writing to a scientific communication tool (academic or traditional transmission). As for the third option, it could be defined as *becoming* a writer based on the conviction that only fictional writing can transmit the uniqueness of the oral exchange as experienced in the analytic process.

Although this is only a brief outline of these options, it would be useful to point out what they have in common. If they are adopted too *innocently*, each one risks being only something to do, as an act of avoidance or disavowal when faced with a disquieting return of the repressed which requires that the analyst experience the loss, the recovery and the acquisition of his "I" in the offer of transference and in transference. Here, avoidance and disavowal are the exact opposite of Freud's creative repression in his process of creating, his essential need to write, and his intrinsic need to build on literature.

For analysts, who continually *refer back* to their experience as analysands, the disquieting return of the repressed is—as it is for everyone—potentially a return of the uncanny, with its most personal motifs, always referring back to the thousand and one intersections of the question of origins with the primal scene, and the primal scene with undetermined substitutes for castration anxiety. Something can only be seen by the subject indirectly, through displacement or reflection, on the condition that he slips away. And if he leaves, undone, whatever the representation or the perception may be, is there something in him that he can only bear to see from the outside, or is he facing something external to him? Is it he who is looking at himself or is he seen by someone else?

The disquieting return of the uncanny might concern the analyst himself at another level. Could it be in relation to transference displaced onto the written corpus of Freudian thought as "subject supposed to know"? In this sense, Freud's initial absence from himself, which he claims to have been central to the invention of psychoanalysis, could become in hindsight, for analysts, the unthinkable scene of a double exclusion (that of Freud and of every analyst individually), bringing loss into the present, as the melancholic threat of a disappearance, foreseen from the start.

The unthinkable would then be reinforced by the Freudian transference to writing, as well as by Freud's envy of writers, who were seen as knowing how to deal better, and even coexist better, with repression; in any case, they were supposed to know better how to make it imaginable to the reader. In fact, whether it be by means of creative transference to writing or envious transference to writers, in this context Freud appears dispossessed of himself. Analysts could face the danger of being reduced to custodians of the supposed knowledge of writers and the supposed knowledge found in creative writing—custodians of psychoanalytic writing and no longer of psychoanalysis.

In other words, in the eyes of psychoanalysts, there can be no intimate relation between creative repression in the invention of psychoanalysis and creative repression in writers. Or, to be more exact, such a relation would reveal a disquieting familiarity to exist between the literary space and the analytic space; the continuity—albeit relative—of one or the other would threaten the identity of psychoanalysis in the eyes of each analyst, endangering the identificatory power of transference to Freud.

Thus, the omission of Goethe's statement and the analysts' loyalty to this omission could be considered the result of Freud's envy of writers, secretly passed down to his heirs and introjected or incorporated by them. This Freudian envy grants a special place to the tutelary figure of Goethe, poet, autobiographer, and investigator, given his *elective affinities* with Freud's passion for writing.[7]

It seems, then, that the intersection of psychoanalysis and writing could constitute a threat to the *sense of identity* of psychoanalysis, the more disturbing for the psychoanalyst since he is left to face alone the affiliation-based divisions fragmenting psychoanalysis. Therefore, this threat must be eliminated at all costs: by the avoidance of the first person in writing, or the avoidance of all writing; by the inflation of the "I" in the constitution of the self as a writer, or the erasure of the "I" in the reduction of literary texts to an excuse (pre-text) for interpretation, that is, ready-made thinking.

Of course, not all writers are the same, including from the limited viewpoint of Freudian identifications. Thus, Goethe is not Sophocles and Schnitzler is not Shakespeare. In other words, Goethe cannot be reduced to an Oedipal figure or a reference to a Greek tragedy, any more than Schnitzler can be reduced to the figure of a double alluding to the ghost inhabiting Hamlet's world.

It is not by chance that the theory of the uncanny was formulated in 1919, at a time of great internal precarity for Freud due to the effects of the war and, more intimately, to the ongoing revision of his metapsychology.

At the metapsychological level, the question of trauma in particular has continued to haunt Freud persistently since the *Wolf Man*. As it has often been pointed out with good reason, the difficulty lies in theorising the uncanny without reducing it to affect: how to think about that which returns, in theory as well as in the mental process under consideration? Is it a repressed representation? Is it an outdated thought? Is it repetition falling short of the pleasure principle? In any case, the question of the traumatic[8] arises, whether the affect associated with the uncanny is seen as a return of the repressed, or as a temporary reinvestment of a previous process.

In addition to metapsychological considerations, it is not by chance that the theory of the uncanny is associated with a writer—E.T.A. Hoffmann—and particularly with the idea that writing is better able than life to call forth the uncanny, since writing reveals language, bringing absence into the present.

* * *

Could it be that, aside from facing insoluble problems of translation, we must distinguish the radically strange from the uncanny? Might it not be truly desirable that the strangeness of home, the *Heimlich*, should offer sufficient resistance to the need to inhabit the internal space peacefully? What if eliminating the strangeness of the home has the potential of threatening the subject with disappearance?

Could the uncanny not consist in being deprived of the fear of becoming lost in the separation of the self from oneself, a separation linked to the internal perception provided by words? Could it not be a feeling of possible disappearance through absence, in the common human experience of being seen by what one sees?[9] In conclusion, we must of course refer to Freud's famous letter to Schnitzler, dated 14 May 1922:

> I think I have avoided you from a kind of reluctance to meet my double. Not that I am easily inclined to identify myself with another, or that I mean to overlook the difference in talent that separates me from you, but whenever I get deeply absorbed in your beautiful creations I invariably seem to find beneath their poetic surface the very presuppositions, interests and conclusions which I know to be my own ... all this moves me with an uncanny feeling of familiarity ... I have gained the impression that you have learned through intuition—though actually as a result of sensitive introspection—everything that I have had to unearth by laborious work on other persons.[10]

Notes

1 Freud, S., *An Outline of Psycho-Analysis*, Wilder Publications, 2010.
2 My attention was drawn to this by a remark made by Janine Altounian.
3 Goethe, J.-W., *Faust, A Tragedy*, Greenberg, M. (Trans.), Yale University Press, 1992.
4 Chiantaretto, J.-F., *De l'acte autobiographique*, Champ Vallon, 1993.
5 See Pontalis, J.-B., *La Force d'attraction*, Seuil, 1990, p. 99.
6 In the sense that with each patient, and even in each session, one has to *become* a psychoanalyst rather than *be* one.
7 Goethe's name was given to the literary prize awarded to Freud's work in 1930.
8 In the sense of contact with the traumatic element.
9 I owe the inspiration for this expression to Didi-Huberman, G., *Ce que nous voyons, ce qui nous regarde* (What We See Looks Back at Us), Éditions de Minuit, 1992.
10 *Letters of Sigmund Freud*, Freud, Ernst L. (Ed.), Dover Publications, 1992.

Chapter 2

The Original, the Originary

The *origins of psychoanalysis*: the phrase is equivocal and expresses a general ambiguity among analysts in regard to the concept of a "primal" scene, a scene which is, in fact, not originary but *original*. This ambiguity takes us back to Freud's hesitation— original, *stricto senso*—in the *Wolf Man*, where he explains the concept of a primal scene, which would soon become the central element of the theory of unconscious phantasy. Could it be that the hesitation at the origins of the originary scene *reveals* the self-generation phantasy present at the start of psychoanalysis?

His desire to prove the relevance of this concept and to distinguish himself from Jung and his "repressive creation" concept led Freud to reduce the originary scene to the witnessing of parental relations, direct or indirect (coupling of animals, for example): a scene considered crucial in the infantile development of the subject, as an event that can be isolated in a historical reconstruction.[1] The distinction between the actual experience of observing the sexual scene and its aftermath—whose metapsychological sense was fully developed by Laplanche and Pontalis[2]—is not only insufficient, but also masks *the* scene, which is strangely absent or ignored.

The scene: the subject as witness to his conception. This definition of the primal scene is evasive, in its phantasmatically structural aspect, structurally undated. There is confusion between the originary scene and the register of the original, between the phantasmatic scene at its beginnings, from its conception to its birth and its psychic construction—a register that is, indefinitely, the source of a prehistoric past indefinitely redefinable.

The subject as witness to his conception: this complete definition of the primal scene is not explicitly acted out in the case of the *Wolf Man*[3]—and is never really acted out. But it is literally displayed in the text written at the same time, and presented by Freud as part of an anti-Jungian dyad, with *On the History of the Psycho-Analytic Movement*.[4] In this text, Freud claims unreservedly and for all time the exclusive place of witness to the conception *in him and by him* of psychoanalysis, that is, his dual *conception* of psychoanalysis and of himself as the first psychoanalyst. Freud sees himself as the only person entitled to define psychoanalysis, and above all to define who is a psychoanalyst and who is not. From this place which is definitely that of the lone creator[5] of psychoanalysis,

DOI: 10.4324/9781003542483-3

who definitely has no other analyst than (the writing of) psychoanalysis, Freud presents himself doubly as the *subject* of his action: subject of its conception and subject of his testimony.

* * *

What are we to do with this self-presentation at the origins of psychoanalysis?[6] Specifically, what can we, as analysts, do with writing itself, writing as the voice of Freud, who created psychoanalysis by means of writing? Often, our view of this question is biased owing to the *originary phantasy* of Freud as a writer, of a Freud whose genius allowed him to make psychoanalysis and writing coincide, founding psychoanalysis on writing and literary creation. As if Freud's founding action had to bring together the first analyst's self-proclamation and the consecration of a writer.

Freud as the writer of psychoanalysis: this phantasy is persistent among analysts, who identify—as if naturally—with Freud's envy of writers, that is, identify through this envy. No doubt, this is particularly noticeable in France, where psychoanalysis was first imported through its texts. However, the problem is that this originary phantasy also reveals something about the origins of psychoanalysis, its creation, the modalities of its construction. It is clear that for Freud there was *original* transference on writing, at the heart of the creative process that gave birth to psychoanalysis.

For analysts to benefit from inheriting this transference on writing, each of them *personally* has to avoid reducing writing to an act of transference, or transference to its depiction in writing—keeping in mind that transference is in great part unconscious and can only be captured in writing fleetingly. That which Freud *laid down* in writing and which allowed him to become an analyst without having an analyst or a supervisor, other analysts must *seek* alone, in the process of becoming analysts, *with or without* their analysts and supervisors, relying on their theoretical references and affiliations.

Becoming an analyst is constantly reformulated through the unique and presumably unprecedented confrontation with each patient. Its transferential character, ungraspable, can nevertheless find expression in writing, *elsewhere*. A psychoanalyst's text, regardless of its form or classification—fiction, essay, theoretico-clinical or metapsychological essay, autobiographical self-presentation—is written and read within a double context: the treatment and what lies outside the treatment. The elsewhere involved here refers more specifically to the analyst's personal ability to withstand not only the strangeness of the analysand's transference, but also the strangeness of his own, which refers back to his transferential "history" as an analysand. The analyst's writing very likely offers him the tenuous, unstable possibility of attesting to his personal effort to achieve a double distancing: from the patients' transferential attributions, and from the transferential presumptions of his own analysis, in principle still ongoing, whether actively pursued or not.

This suggests the possibility of transference stemming from a transferential offer made by the analyst, before the analysand's transference and the analyst's countertransference: an offer *of* transference. To discuss the function of writing for the analyst, beyond the formal diversity and the absolute singularity of personal investments, it appears to be necessary to reconsider the question of Freud's transference onto writing: no longer the writing of psychoanalysis, but more specifically the writing of a "history of the origin" of psychoanalysis. I see a need to reconsider, based on the Freudian account of the origins, the founding account given in two segments: *The History of the Psychoanalytic Movement* (1917) and *An Autobiographical Study* (1925).

This account closely intertwines the originary scene of the conception of psychoanalysis—in Freud's mind as well as without Freud, but structured by him in such a way as to allow us to (re)construct it for him—and the original register of the birth of psychoanalysis. Someone is called to testify—Freud—who cannot be present but will be partially represented by a witness—Freud!—who will only be able to testify regarding a portion of the object examined ... before his future witnesses: the psychoanalysts who are Freud's heirs. This testimonial saturation contained in the writing is likely to clarify the phantasy function of Freud, the writer. Analysts are placed in a position to conceptualise—as his successors and therefore differently from Freud—transference *in* the writing, rather than transference *onto* writing. They do this hoping—or expecting?—to identify that which the analyst's writing has in common with that of historians, despite their distinctly different approaches, in terms of affinity with the poets: the work of providing *intimate* testimony about the relation between internal interlocution and interlocution, speaking to oneself and speaking, what words cannot convey and what lies beyond words, the secret as a condition of speech, and the fate of the secret in writing.

> We need history because we need to rest. A respite is needed to rest our consciousness, so that the possibility of consciousness continues to exist—not only the seat of thought, but of practical reasoning which gives full latitude to act. Saving the past, saving time from the frenzy of the present: this is what poets do meticulously. You have to be willing to be less strong, to be idle, to defuse the endangering of temporality which wreaks havoc on experience and scorns childhood.[7]

* * *

The psychoanalysts' "need for history" reflects their legitimate wish to have a respite from Freud's claim of writing the history of the origins of psychoanalysis—a task that troubled Freud at the time of his difficult conceptualisation of the primal scene with the *Wolf Man*, and has continued to trouble psychoanalysts ever since. Insisting on what he considers a historically oriented reconstruction, Freud is unable to present the scene clearly: the subject as witness to his conception. The scene remains blurred, never acquiring definition as a strictly phantasmatic scene without temporality because, in *The History of the Psychoanalytic Movement*, its conceptualisation takes place within the supposedly historical reconstitution of the writing of the "genesis of psychoanalysis." As if the creation of the primal scene concept cannot be distinguished from the scene of the conception of psychoanalysis, a scene of the origins (re)constructed by Freud and presented to his successors as an originary scene.

Freud presents the case of the *Wolf Man* as a supplement to a "polemic of a personal character"[8] directed against Jung by means of a text he considers a historical account. The confusion in the text and in its different registers is literally incredible, as can be seen in the assertion of the objectivity of psychoanalytic facts and the supposedly biographical demonstration of the primal scene. This shows how biased the conceptualisation of the primal scene is, due to the break with Jung: only one perspective is *authorised*, and lays the ground for the origins (of the concept) of a primal scene, as well as the origins of psychoanalysis.

> If in what follows I bring any contribution to the history of the psychoanalytic movement nobody must be surprised at the subjective nature of this paper, nor at the role which falls to me therein. For psychoanalysis is my creation; for ten years I was the only one occupied with it ... Even today, when I am no longer the only psychoanalyst, I feel myself justified in assuming that none can know better than myself what psychoanalysis is, wherein it differs from other methods of investigating the psychic life, what its name should cover, or what might better be designated as something else.[9]

Thus, this *impossible* perspective structures the confusion between the originary scene and the *register* of the originary, a confusion often seen among psychoanalysts, particularly when they write and thereby consent to giving a readable account of their relationships with the origins: with the Freudian corpus, that is, a corpus always written as ongoing writing, *always unfinished and always holding the potential of creating psychoanalysts*.

The Freudian corpus is not solely the place where Freud's thought was formulated and developed, but also the place where he enacted a phantasy of self-generation. This phantasy can be said to have been confirmed retroactively by the Freudian oeuvre's power of continued generation: by the legitimation it offers to psychoanalysts and their associations—since the Freudian corpus has been considered, generation after generation, and despite repeated divisions, that which safeguards the status "psychoanalyst" and legitimates its use. This is where Freud did not think through *to its conclusion* the primal scene he portrayed in writing as a phantasy of self-generation in his 1914 text: an exclusive testimony to the creation *by him alone* of psychoanalysis, specifically, of his coming into being as the first psychoanalyst—*that is*, the creator of his creation. Self-presentation was going to testify to the miracle of self-generation even more explicitly in 1925 than it had in 1914.

> While I was writing my "History of the Psycho-Analytic Movement" in 1914, there recurred to my mind some remarks that had been made to me by Breuer, Charcot, and Chrobak, which might have led me to this discovery earlier. But at the time I heard them I did not understand what these authorities meant; indeed, they had told me more than they knew themselves or were prepared to defend. What I heard from them lay dormant and inactive within me, until the chance of my cathartic experiments brought it out as an apparently original discovery.[10]

Freud is saying: the conception of psychoanalysis can only be attributed to the fertilisation of ovules implanted and carried to term within me, Freud; it is the transmission and insemination of a secret, with its secret progression in me. The only legitimate witness, who can certify to the facts, which are diverse by nature[11]—historical, scientific, and personal at the same time—is I myself, Freud. *I, Freud*: a witness made absent to himself, who can only testify based on the re-constitution of his absence and the absence of those who planted in him the seeds of their unsuspected knowledge. Thus, biographers and successors will have to follow the only possible path: *my presentation of the facts—in other words, they will have to trust what I say*.

What can we do with this legacy, this obscure discourse on discourse, this presentation of the origins laid down forever as the source of the successors' originary phantasies? There is no doubt that, for psychoanalysts, recourse to writing can constitute an answer.

* * *

Is it not the case that freeing oneself from Freud's imaginary power by desisting from being an analyst or a writer *for* him means accepting your own unprecedented position as interpreter, and creating the possibility of testifying in and through writing, *elsewhere*? Would analysts not do well to avail themselves of a space of writing, in a relationship imbued with the same strange familiarity as that present in psychoanalytic treatment? This relationship is tied intimately enough to the transferential material between patient and analyst, and sufficiently unrelated to it, to belong to neither of them, nor to both at the same time.

Neither analyst nor writer: to act neither as Freud's analyst, in the role of the analyst of one's analysts, nor as a writer in Freud's place, thereby abandoning the possibility of writing rooted in the analysis—which is the inevitable specificity of the analyst's writing, whether this writing refers to analytic work or not.

What is to be done with Freud's envy of writers, personified best and most painfully by Schnitzler? This envy of Freud's is processed in many and varied ways by analysts who write. But in France two major figures stand out when it comes to shedding light on what is at stake when an analyst turns to writing: Jean-Bertrand Pontalis and Didier Anzieu. Beyond the importance of these two giants of contemporary psychoanalysis, whose theoretical works include texts on writing, we can point out the iconic value of *Love of Beginnings* and *Beckett et le psychanalyste*, considered as important works in their own right, independently of the overall psychoanalytic and literary oeuvre of their authors, and regardless of how they differ.

While Pontalis has produced a considerable number of literary works,[12] this is not the case for Anzieu: he describes his two "literary" works[13] as the writing of an analyst, not that of a writer. This difference proves to be significant and likely to make it possible for the analyst to choose two modes of investing writing, distinct enough to answer even today's needs in a context where, more than ever, analysts seek a personal manner of writing. Indeed, Anzieu's two books reproduce in two opposite forms the autobiographical perspective of Freud's self-presentation.

First, *Love of Beginnings*. This autobiographical work explicitly focuses on the writing of origins, written by an author whose contributions deal with the theory of the originary, deliberately omits to discuss the question of the analyst-in-the-making. Instead, it designates words as an object in common, tying together the analyst, the writer, the editor and the translator:

> I practice psychoanalysis, I edit books and a journal, I read manuscripts, I write from time to time, sometimes I translate. More than most, here I am, a man busy in different spheres with the same object: words.[14]

Psychoanalysis is only invoked through a brief reference to Lacan, without a context, in an eminently Sartrian tone: Pontalis claims to have left him to avoid succumbing to the influence of his teaching.[15] In truth, the figure exerting his influence on the narrator is Sartre. He is very present in Pontalis' account which, although critical, makes clear the latter's elective admiration, "because he too was a writer."[16] Above all, Sartre is implicitly present as a reference figure for writing, as the one who created a *certain* manner of investing the "flesh" of words.

> That the word became flesh is decidedly the only thing that interests me. In my view, the mystery of incarnation is not a religious, but rather an esthetic question.[17]

The power of embodiment exerted by language is, in fact, a recurring theme in all of Pontalis' work, from fictional texts to essays. This theme is worthy of specific study, quite apart from the reference to Sartre. In the text cited here, several passages reveal identification with Sartre, particularly with the impossible mourning for the prematurely deceased father, but above all with the obsession concerning the immobilisation of the body by language:

> What I always fear is to be reduced to a present that offers nothing, a mute present—mute like an identity card, like a tombstone. Words kill when they designate us.[18]

We might be reading something out of *Being and Nothingness* or *The Words*! When Pontalis declares "love and hatred of words"[19] to be the theme of his book, asserting that they govern all investment in objects, he places himself in a phantasmatic Sartrian lineage, regardless of his break with Sartre and with *Les Temps modernes*, precisely over the question of psychoanalysis. I suggest that *Love of Beginnings* be read as a narrative determined by identification with the author of *The Words*, indissociable from counter-identification with Freud's envy of writers. In this respect, Pontalis' book could be said to be the contrary of *An Autobiographical Study*. Although both texts are intended to be autobiographical accounts substituting beginnings for future developments, the authors follow inverse paths to accomplish their aims.

Freud's founding account, deliberately free of autobiographical substance, is written to relate the construction of psychoanalysis and to assert that the author was its creator and the first analyst. Both the form and the content illustrate that Freud forgoes writing as a writer—and therefore relinquishes the power he envies. By contrast, Pontalis' account, deliberately written to testify to the bodily sources and substance of words, intends to confirm the author's status as a writer. Moreover, it claims a fundamental convergence of his roles as analyst and writer.

It is not the writing of the analyst and the author which converge, but that which incites the author to write and the analyst to speak in his clinical practice. It is as if the writer is better able than the analyst to testify in writing about the analytic process, outside the framework of the treatment. *I, Pontalis, disciple of The Words, I shall (could) be the writer of psychoanalysis*, not in the sense of writing it, but in the sense of being the writer that the founder of psychoanalysis could not be. Phantasy work—the expression is welcome here—can be defined as follows: to fulfil Freud's desire regarding the illustrative power of the work of the writer's unconscious—work of which he is unaware—to embody its object by becoming a writer.[20]

Didier Anzieu's book is quite different. *Beckett et le psychanalyste* undertakes to continue the written account of Freud's self-analysis. Autobiography as self-obituary: the parody presented in *Contes à rebours*[21] takes the form of writing that shifts from self-analysis to writing *on behalf* of another: first Freud, then Beckett.[22] The autobiographer writes about his life from his position beyond life, although this position poses a threat to the son of Lacan's Aimée: that of slipping into the role of one who is dead: identifying with the dead child in the mother who is dead to herself. But when writing an account of the self-analysis of the other, slipping into the role of the one who is dead gives the writing the power to free itself of the incorporation of the dead child in the mother, to come to life in the other, and thus to phantasmatically restore the mother's power to live.

What Anzieu intends to do in *Beckett et le psychanalyste* is to make readable, by writing it, the "self-analysis by means of literary creation" undertaken by Beckett in the first part of his oeuvre (1946 to 1960). This self-analysis is considered an elaboration in the aftermath of the analysis with Bion, prematurely interrupted and referencing Bion's own self-analysis, conducted through his theoretical research, with a parallel elaborative objective.

Anzieu divides his book into two parts: a diary bearing the dates of the reading of Beckett, followed by self-analytic commentary. This double narrative portrays writing taking place *between* Beckett and Bion, thereby revealing the unprecedented locus of writing: the space between identification with the writer and identification by psychoanalysis. And this new space of writing frees Anzieu from his assignment to the place of the son of the living-dead Aimée, an impossible position between identification with his mother and the identification made by Lacan—the mother's psychiatrist *and* the son's psychoanalyst.

* * *

The question we must answer is: in order for the analyst to find a writing stance likely to *be enriched* by the experience of words emerging at the intersection of the analysand's and the analyst's unconscious, does the latter have to consent to become a writer, or consent to give this up? In either case, the consent would have the same aim: to create an unprecedented mode of self-presentation, which would allow desirable free-flowing communication between the two poles.

The two-in-one text Anzieu produces by dividing the narrative illustrates very clearly how writing can testify to the internal alterity of the analyst at work—from a place beyond the analytic situation, exerting its effect on this situation through the analyst's internal interlocution. The place beyond can be related, first of all, to the distance between the frame and the analyst, between the person of the analyst and the analyst as interpreter, and between the multiple positions of the transitional object held by the patient and the position of subject of a transference reserved for oneself through various means.

The distance is provided by the analyst's thinking process, which should establish a vital relation between the "frame of mind of the man who is reflecting" and that of "a man who is observing his own psychical processes," to refer back to a remark Freud made in *The Interpretation of Dreams*,[23] from a different perspective. This vital relation between thinking and self-observation could be described as the pleasure of thinking in context: the pleasure of investigating one's psychic functioning, which prompts the analysand's investigation of his own functioning, whose interpretation and *reinterpretation* are transformative.

This illustrates a fundamental aspect of the asymmetry between the analyst and the analysand, which ensures that the analyst's internal alterity will serve the needs of the analytic process, and reinforce the thirdness inherent in the frame. The analyst's internal alterity is placed *at* the service of the process, but is mobilised into action by the internal experience of his listening, of his experience of being listened to, and his ability to express himself in the words which come to his mind, whether they produce speech addressed to someone or not.

This internal experience, which owes its specificity to the patient's transferential solicitation, could serve as the definition of the analyst's internal interlocution, from the perspective opened by the idea of an internal witness—the function held by the different figures of the other in oneself, which allow the subject to glimpse himself in his interaction with words, in the continuity of his psychic functioning. This makes it possible to prefigure the possibility for the analyst in the session to experience a discrepancy between his countertransferential affects and his transference—an ever-present possibility in the analytic process.

It is here that the analyst's transference brings to mind the impossible aspect of the Freud/Ferenczi relation, creating significant confusion between the absence of an analyst for the founder of psychoanalysis, and the undeniable fallibility of the analysis of the man who started it over, aspiring to give it a new foundation. This confusion creates a transferential scene at once original and originary for each analyst. The original scene refers back to the beginnings of the psychoanalysis to which Freud claims to be the only one who can testify. And an originary scene referring back to new starts rekindled by that which each analyst establishes as he secretly listens to his listening[24]—or, to say it differently, by the "potential writing" allowing the analyst to access the resistances of his transference.

This term refers to one of the registers of the analyst's thinking process in the session, opening a perspective that makes it possible to go beyond the patient's transferential reactions: a viewpoint creating a distance from the transferential function. Potential writing fitting this definition is inseparable from the elaboration of countertransference and from the analyst's own transference.

When the analyst writes, prompted by the request for an analysis or by an element external to the treatment, is it not the case that his writing testifies *in retrospect*, between the known and the unknown, to the creativity associated with this premise? Does it not testify, in the intimacy of the space between them, to the good and bad encounters of each party's transferences, from a perspective supporting the transferential offer of transference made by the analyst—and thus, asymmetrical?

Writing may also enable the analyst to imagine what became, in his own psyche, of that which had resisted analysis in his analyst(s), based on his own resistances in his transference to his patients. Could it be that writing allows these unanalysed elements, now belonging to no one, to be partially forgotten in the verve of creativity? Could writing allow creative repression, the token and signature of a style which appears as a manifestation of the being—not one of his possessions or attributes—sufficiently free of the obligations and constraints associated with the inevitable logic of belonging?

* * *

Freud's position is absolutely unique, since writing allows his thought to unfold simultaneously in the inner space of internal interlocution and in the public space where the reader is asked to witness an ongoing thinking process. After Freud, psychoanalysts must recognise, uneasily, that all theorising is elaborated through self-theorising, which is by nature fallible, though necessary. No doubt we could even say that analysts can only acquire knowledge if they admit this, that they can only attain creativity through confrontation with this fallibility. The latter points to a structural fact: the analyst's thinking process in and outside the analytic setting is sustained by the elaboration of the countertransference. This in turn is subjected to the effect of the analyst's transference, at the heart of which there is the one not yet analysed, prompted to act in a singular manner with each patient, but always in a manner related to the transformation by the analyst of what was left unanalysed in his own analyst(s).

Here, the analyst's transference confronts him, not with the act of creating or even with Freud's creation, but with the temptation to imitate the Freudian transgression: self-presentation as the presentation of a subject totally and definitively in possession of his act, subject of its *conception* and subject in the act of testifying to it.

From the perspective of psychoanalysts in their setting, the self-generation phantasy laid out in the Freudian self-presentation acquires, at least in latent form, the value of a transgression of the limits of the knowable, with the assertion of full knowledge of oneself and perfect convergence of the self with one's self-representation.[25] At the origins of psychoanalysis, a transgression acted as a temptation, literally producing a primal scene shared by all analysts.

To transgress means to cross over to the other side. As founder and creator of psychoanalysis, Freud can only transgress by claiming for himself the place of the analyst which he could neither have nor be—by elaborating psychoanalysis in writing and describing the founding process of self-presentation. And analysts are left with the transgressive temptation of becoming Freud's analysts, which they must acknowledge in order to escape it. They can either confront Freudian transgression by thinking it through, or give in to the temptation of becoming Freud's analysts in order to avoid awareness of the inevitable temptation of holding the place of the analyst of one's analyst: this is the alternative left to every analyst after Freud.

This place obliterated by Freud must be left vacant, and each analyst must question for himself what it reveals about the temptation to become the analyst of one's analyst.

This is where the Freud-Ferenczi relation is relevant: in the original starting over of psychoanalysis. Freud, as the founder who wishes to remain in possession of his oeuvre in order to ensure its transmissibility, is forced to remain an unanalysable analyst, having had no analyst other than the creative process of psychoanalysis. Ferenczi, opposite him, is also forced to become an unanalysable analyst due to the unavoidable lack of an analyst for Freud, *his inexorable lack of experience as an analysand.* An unanalysable analyst for whom the theory—at the level of renewal of metapsychology—corresponds to a desperate effort to create an analyst for Freud, in hopes of finally benefitting from him as analysable analyst and analysand. *Trapped* in their relation, each of them protests against what is unknowable in the transference, and at the same time against the experience of the unknowable in the transference. But, while the endless beginnings of psychoanalysis had already separated Freud and Ferenczi repeatedly, giving it a new start forced Ferenczi more and more into inescapable separation.

Psychoanalysts are left to inherit not only Freud's internal dialogue, but *also* the impossible but creative dialogue between Freud and Ferenczi. They claim this inheritance by recourse to questioning concerning their own psychic functioning, as their patients reveal it. This questioning brings the analyst in contact with the unknowable: the unconscious and its sources.

* * *

We are dealing with the desire to know and its relation to transgression, which Piera Aulagnier theorised with great clarity:

> The desire to know will trip over its own structure, which demands that the subject only be able to hold his position as desiring subject (desiring to know) through constant transgression of the known in search of an inexhaustible unknown, the last form taken by the various manifestations of castration, the last reminder of the required renouncing of the omnipotence of a desire that always wants to name the object-cause of its emergence.[26]

This cannot fail to bring to mind the paradoxical injunction in Genesis, in the phrasing of the first Law, which associates the prohibition with its anticipated transgression, and even spells out the corresponding sanction: "You may freely eat of every tree of the garden, but of the tree of the knowledge of good and evil, you shall not eat, for in the day that you eat of it you shall surely die."[27]

In the biblical perspective, the eating of knowledge, as an act where eating and knowing are indistinguishable, asserts the primacy of the gaze, expressed in the seductive and manipulative (in this context: perverse) words of the serpent, which lead to transgression *and* knowledge: "they knew that they were naked"[28]— formulated using the Hebrew verb *laddat*,[29] which in the biblical text always refers to both the act of knowing and the sexual act.

Beyond this biblical resonance, Aulagnier's perspective is completely Freudian, pursuing the path laid out in *Three Essays on the Theory of Sexuality*.[30] The object of knowledge is the sexual, in a sexual context; knowledge is sexual by nature, given its autoerotic sources.[31] This assertion makes it possible to conceive of the unknowable as doubly inherent to knowledge. The unknowable aspect of his conception exposes the subject to an originary exclusion to which phantasmatic activity supporting the primal scene is expected to testify by default and for life. Moreover, the unknowable inherent to his psychic structuring, under the constraints of castration and lack, exposes the subject to his original infantile dependence.

The vital dependence of the *infans* is indissociably an aspect of self-preservation and autoeroticism, given that the latter is determined by a pleasure of functioning gained in the experience of having been the source of sexual and narcissistic gratification for the primordial other, at the stage of vital need satisfaction. The sources of this pleasure of functioning, fundamental to acceptance of life in the Ferenczian perspective,[32] are unknowable. Just as, in the Winnicottian perspective, the sources of a feeling of continuity of being, and of the true self as the support of creative autoeroticism, are unknowable.

The metapsychological contribution made by Aulagnier—the theoretician of fundamental violence—proves to be essential in the exploration of this second aspect of the unknowable within knowledge, from the standpoint of the original pleasure taken by the psyche in experiencing itself in the investment made by the primordial other. The messenger function of the maternal psyche establishes an ideational representation serving to store and safeguard a knowledge of the being of the subject as he is being constructed, which identifies the *infans* and to which he identifies. The subject has no access to this knowledge. It designates the unknowable as a-topical, a place without place, a place designated only by a negative, a *forbidden* place: off limits to the future words of the *infans*, but meant to be stated in the silence between words and within each word.

In Aulagnier's view, the unknowable is the process constituting the *infans* in the identificatory and identifying attribution made by the maternal psyche: primary violence and its anticipatory *power*. In other words, the unknowable originates in the repression process inherent to the activity of the maternal psyche in its sexual and narcissistic investment of the *infans*. The unknowable determines the nature of feelings, which brings about the nomination of affects and "the interpretation connecting an unknowable sensation with a cause supposedly suited to what is experienced."[33]

The unknowable at the heart of knowledge designates both originary knowledge and its origin, that is, the foundation of the "I" as the subject of knowing, in a double anchoring of the desire to know. This double anchoring culminates in the emergence of the speaking subject. It could be associated with the primal scene, in which and through which the subject constructs his fate throughout his life, by acting as the subject of his phantasies; as well as with the original interpretation of the maternal psyche, in which and through whose transformations, the subject becomes the subject of his thoughts. Between the primal scene and the original interpretation, there is perhaps the element Freud seemed to allude to in *An Outline of Psychoanalysis*, the confidence of the baby in the mother's return, beyond his hope: a surplus of *confidence*, which could be considered the necessary condition for the desire to know.

In any case, the enigma of the shaping of the human subject by the psyche of another includes a distance between the initial inscription of an experience and its representation. This distance is due to the constitution of the infant's psyche through the investment made by the maternal psyche in the thinking process, which inscribes an excess, so that meaning is not an object of knowledge. In other words, in order to see and to see oneself, one has to have been held in someone's gaze and then lost this original gaze—a lost gaze which remains partially present and is to be found again in the excess in the gaze of a current other.

The unknowable implies an inalterable double loss: the mother and the maternal psyche. The mother is called elsewhere by her desire—an elsewhere that inscribes in the infant the mark of externality, which opens onto the dimension of the internal alterity of the other as the announcement of the oedipal third: the other of the other. The maternal psyche, as the locus of desiring interpretation, is to be invested in phantasy as an *inaccessible and desirable source of desire*. This double loss, necessarily enigmatic,[34] constitutes the source of the desire for knowledge, taking the form of a "desire of knowledge about desire."[35]

This is also where, in the absence of a pathological impediment, loss is believed to pre-inscribe prohibition: of knowledge about one's desire to know, and of knowledge about the desire of the other. To know implies acceptance of the separation between knowledge and jouissance—the latter resulting from the limitless assimilation of knowledge and pleasure. Ultimately, what must be accepted is the inherent gap between representation and the represented, between experience and the representable, between pleasure and jouissance. This is the condition for gaining access to the I, since it designates the subject as subject of his phantasies and thoughts: subject of that which divides him. Becoming the subject of his thinking requires thinking with pleasure and submitting this pleasure to thought.[36]

* * *

The desire to know underlies all analytic treatment, since the latter is the creation by two people of a work of reflection that specifically elicits the "mutual dependence"[37] involved in any relation: a joint creation, by the analysand and the analyst, together and separately, of thoughts that are a source of pleasure because they are unprecedented. The desire to know is at the origins of psychoanalysis as well because in its very nature, and in the creative process, there is a duality, in the double sense of a creative duality and a confrontation likely to lead to murder. This confrontation, by revealing its murderous potential in the impossible *analytic relation* between Freud and Ferenczi, brings to light the transgression at the Freudian foundation.

Freud, the creator of psychoanalysis, who created the psychoanalyst in the internal dialogue carried on through writing and through his appeal to his successors to witness his construction, held the obliterated place of the analyst's analyst, for himself and for all the analysts he trained, *starting with* Ferenczi. There would never be an analyst for the man who, irrevocably alone, became an analyst by inventing psychoanalysis for all future analysts. Thus, there would never be a teaching analyst for Ferenczi's analyst, nor an analyst trained for him.

Freud's endeavour, at the beginnings of psychoanalysis, to occupy all places while he enacted a self-generating phantasy determined Ferenczi to attempt to hold his own place as an analyst. This in itself is an attack on the very idea of internal dialogue, within each analyst and between the analysand and the analyst; a questioning of the internal experience of the unknowable supposedly triggered by the analyst's transference.

But is it not each analyst's personal responsibility to forgo occupying his analyst's place—as analyst and as analysand—and to transform this symboligenic vacancy into a vital and uncertain source of psychoanalytic knowledge? We would then be well advised to re-examine what took place between Freud and Ferenczi in order to clarify what takes place again and again for each analyst: the revision of the new beginnings of psychoanalysis by the Freudian beginnings … and not only the contrary.

Notes

1 The reading of the *Wolf Man* in parallel with Freud's founding text, presented in these pages, was developed in Chiantaretto, J.-F., *De l'acte autobiographique*, Champ Vallon, 1993.
2 Laplanche, J. and Pontalis, J.-B., *Fantasme originaire: Fantasmes des origines, origines du fantasme*, Hachette, 1985.
3 Freud, S., *From the History of an Infantile Neurosis*, S.E. 17, Hogarth.
4 Freud, S., *On the History of the Psycho-Analytic Movement*, S.E. 14, Hogarth.
5 Until 1906 or 1907, as he stated in 1925, in Freud, S., *An Autobiographical Study*, S.E. 20, Hogarth.
6 Self-presentation as a posture is present in most of Freud's texts; Freud plays the role of "historian of the creation" of psychoanalysis, and witness—who asks the reader to be witness—to a developing thought process which constantly reconsiders itself. But *On the History of the Psycho-Analytic Movement* and *An Autobiographical Study* radicalise the historian's act, making it the subject of discussion and asserting that it is the exclusive sign and attribute of the founding act.
7 Boucheron, P., *Ce que peut l'histoire*, Fayard, 2016 (TN: my translation).
8 Freud, S., *From the History of an Infantile Neurosis*, S.E. 17, Hogarth.
9 Freud, S., *On the History of the Psycho-Analytic Movement*, S.E. 14, Hogarth.
10 Freud, S., *An Autobiographical Study*, S.E. 20, Hogarth, p. 24.
11 Rey, J.-M., "Freud et l'écriture de l'histoire," *L'Écrit du temps*, 6, 1984.
12 In addition to his editorial work, which has contributed greatly to establishing a new and durable distinction between the analyst's writing and the writing of psychoanalysis.
13 Anzieu, D., *Contes à rebours*, Clancier-Guénaud, 1987; Anzieu, D., *Beckett et le psychanalyste*, Mentha, 1992.
14 Pontalis, J.-B., *Love of Beginnings*, Free Association Books, 1993.
15 Pontalis, J.-B., *Love of Beginnings*, Free Association Books, 1993.
16 Pontalis, J.-B., *Love of Beginnings*, Free Association Books, 1993.
17 Pontalis, J.-B., *Love of Beginnings*, Free Association Books, 1993.
18 Pontalis, J.-B., *Love of Beginnings*, Free Association Books, 1993.
19 Pontalis, J.-B., *Love of Beginnings*, Free Association Books, 1993.
20 My intention is only to put into words the phantasy *secreted* by Pontalis' text—in the sense of a secret displayed and *secreted* by the writing—without reducing all his literary contributions to this text, or the totality of his work to literary texts, or the author himself to his text and to this phantasy …
21 Anzieu, D., "Le nécrologiste," in *Contes à rebours*, Clancier-Guénaud, 1987.
22 For an overview of Anzieu's autobiographical writings, see Chiantaretto, J.-F., *De l'acte autobiographique*, Champ Vallon Éditions, 1998.
23 Freud, S., *The Interpretation of Dreams*, S.E. 4–5, Hogarth.
24 See *infra*.
25 In this respect, Freudian self-presentation, which enacts the autobiographical posture excessively, is in total contrast to psychoanalysis!
26 Aulagnier, P., "Le 'désir de savoir' dans ses rapports à la transgression" (1967), in Bouhsira, J., Dreyfus-Asséo, S., Durieux, M.-C., and Janin, C., *Transgression*, PUF, Monographies et débats de psychanalyse, 2009, pp. 31–48 (TN: my translation).
27 Genesis 2:17.
28 Genesis 3:7.
29 Munk, Rabbi E., *The Call of the Torah*, Mesorah Publications, 2007.
30 Jean Laplanche (1962) changed this faulty translation to *Trois essais sur la théorie sexuelle*.
31 See Chiantaretto, J.-F., "À propos de la première transgression," *Topique*, 92 (3) 2005.

32 Ferenczi, S., "The Unwelcome Child and His Death-Instinct," *International Journal of Psycho-Analysis*, 10, 1929: 125–129.

33 Aulagnier, P., *The Violence of Interpretation*, Sheridan, A. (Trans.), Routledge, 2001.

34 This enigma constitutes the focus and object of the perverse and/or borderline inclination.

35 Aulagnier, P., "Le 'désir de savoir' dans ses rapports à la transgression," in Bouhsira, J., Dreyfus-Asséo, S., Durieux, M.-C., and Janin, C., *Transgression*, PUF, Monographies et débats de psychanalyse, 2009 [1967], p. 47 (TN: my translation).

36 Aulagnier, P., "Le droit au secret: condition pour pouvoir penser" (The Right to Secrecy. A Condition for Thinking), in *Un interprète en quête de sens*, Ramsay, 1986 [1976], pp. 235–237.

37 Aulagnier, P., "Le droit au secret: condition pour pouvoir penser" (The Right to Secrecy. A Condition for Thinking), in *Un interprète en quête de sens*, Ramsay, 1986 [1976], p. 227.

Part 2

Renewing Psychoanalysis

A journey from the beginnings of psychoanalysis—plural in Freud's founding process and in everything that followed—to the beginnings of a psychoanalysis, always plural and unprecedented with each patient … With each analyst, the question of making a new start supposedly arises again. It is considered again from the perspective of the inherent relation between Freud's original transference onto writing, and each analyst's transference in the context of his work—a relation to which the analyst testifies when he writes, intentionally or not. Here, this relation will be examined in light of the new start proposed by Ferenczi,[1] and of the Freud/Ferenczi dialogue—between original and originary—and its transferential effects, the ultimate aim being to elucidate the specificity of borderline practice.

Now and then, at the origins of the construction of psychoanalysis and of the borderline state, the possibility of psychic murder found occasions to deny its own existence in order to succeed (partially) in taking hold. In both cases, the impetus which brings about the analyst's transference also serves to render what took place usable. Render usable: invest the originary event that occurred but took *no place*, and was materialised through transference onto the psychoanalyst, who can mobilise his vital creativity—with and against self-destructiveness—a concept incomparably developed by Winnicott.

Alternatively, we could say that now and then, very differently, of course, murder of creativity came to be *sufficiently* perpetrated because the possibility of psychic murder had not been *sufficiently* thinkable. And, in the aftermath, in the more revealing borderline sphere, it is up to each analyst to make this *possibility* emerge in the transference … so that the already perpetrated murder of thought does not act as the announcement of a future murder.

Note

1 I wish to acknowledge Wladimir Granoff's decisive pioneering work in his reading of Ferenczi, although the notion of starting over I propose here focuses on a different idea than the one implicit in the formulation stating Granoff's position: "Freud invented psychoanalysis [but] it was Ferenczi who put it into practice" (Granoff, W., *Lacan, Ferenczi et Freud*, Gallimard, 2001, p. 85). I would also like to express my thanks to the team of *Coq-Héron*, and particularly to Judith Dupont, its founder and driving spirit. Being part of this journal's Editorial Board (1989–2001) allowed me to make Ferenczi's legacy my own.

DOI: 10.4324/9781003542483-4

Chapter 3

The Ferenczian Renewal[1]

Reflecting on the *affected* thoughts of the analyst, to make the affects in the analysand's words thinkable … Ferenczi was the first to theorise the analyst's thinking in the session. He developed a "metapsychology of the technique,"[2] including a "metapsychology of the analyst's mental processes during analysis."[3] He made this proposal from a unique and unprecedented position.

Ferenczi *starts* psychoanalysis *over*, with and against Freud, building on Freudian foundations—plural, since Freud constantly revised his creation. Ferenczi was the first of those who proposed new beginnings—they, after all, constitute the history of psychoanalysis—and he was the most influential of Freud's interlocutors in the beginnings of psychoanalysis. But most importantly, he took part in the founding process *from the inside*, in a creative dialogue with Freud—undeniably unique and incomparable. Ferenczi is the only analyst other than Freud who personifies the creative duality, the original duality that Freud initially carried alone: *the only one of Freud's interlocutors who could invest and be invested as if he were an internal interlocutor*.

Ferenczi finds and loses himself in a relationship with Freud at the origins of psychoanalysis. He is also at the heart of a primal scene inevitably occurring in the session due to the analyst's position, and which every analyst can presumably render thinkable, if not during, at least after the session. This primal scene solicits a vacant place, the one of an analyst for Freud. This void at the heart of the Freud/Ferenczi relation and at the source of the impossibility of conducting an analysis designates a vacant place which psychoanalysts are inevitably tempted to fill, and which they *must not* fill, in order to transform it, as much as possible, into absence.

The irremediable absence of an analyst for Freud is tied to his successors' willingness—inherent to the position of an analyst—to forgo imagining themselves in the place of their analysts. This place makes it possible to constitute a composite transferential figure: one's analyst or analysts, his supervisors, their analysts, and, consequently, all of the referential figures attesting to a recognised identity. That this place is empty—the consent to leave it empty—makes it possible, on the imaginary plane, to conceive of its transferential consequences. If the place remains *vacant*, it becomes the point of convergence of the work of elaborating the

DOI: 10.4324/9781003542483-5

transferential fantasies which constitute it. There is no doubt that here the vacancy becomes the most reliable indicator of sufficient liberation from the effects of affiliations and of collusions with the patients' fantasies or imagination, themselves directly influenced by the temptation to become the analysts of their analyst.

Refraining from occupying this place, making room for the one who is absent: a question also related to the status of self-analysis in Freud and Ferenczi's case. Strictly speaking, self-analysis can only be recounted in the aftermath, and by another person, as Didier Anzieu did with Freud's, reconstituted from traces in the latter's correspondence and texts. Ferenczi's self-analysis, which he cannot put in writing despite believing this to be possible, is conducted by addressing an absent/ absented analyst, in an impossible attempt at "compensating" this absence by giving psychoanalysis a new start. On the other hand, Freud's self-analysis, which he cannot put into writing despite his belief to the contrary, is conducted by addressing an analyst whose absence is irremediable—an absence that the beginnings of psychoanalysis are charged with compensating.

What place should be given to the analytic aspect of the Freud/Ferenczi relation? Rather, how can we delimit what I would call an intermediary zone between analysis and self-analysis? Or, very specifically, what Ferenczi describes as "a special technique of self-analysis—by letter (that is, with the constant representation of the presence of an analyst)."[4] This formulation clearly expresses the hybrid nature of this self-analytic process with its underlying paradox: self-analysis claiming the status of *self-psychoanalysis*,[5] but requiring self-writing—which naturally plays a part in the reinforcement of repression associated with secondarisation, and serves to allow the absence of the other, while here the mode of address intends to render the other present.

In time, Ferenczi abandoned the illusion that he could be the subject of the written account of his self-analysis. With understandable reluctance, Yves Lugrin advances the hypothesis that Ferenczi's letters to Freud[6] have another-self-analytic function, especially during the period between 1912 and 1919, when self-analysis was most intense and when his three brief sequences of analysis with Freud took place (between 1914 and 1916, a few weeks at a time, but intensively).

How are we to think of the association of this analysis with Ferenczi's self-analysis? Was this an analysis "finished but not terminated," as Freud wrote Ferenczi on 24 October 1916:[7] an analysis in three segments, made possible before, and completed afterwards by self-analysis?[8] Or was it a self-analysis attempting to bring Freud to the position of analyst, and gradually acknowledging the impossibility of the task, given their mutual resistances? Freud, the analyst without an analyst, turns a blind eye to his own transference, and neglects working with Ferenczi's transference. In this situation, Ferenczi is an analyst forced to fall back on self-analysis for lack of analysis, all the while tormented by the temptation to become Freud's analyst, in order to turn him into his own analyst. From this point of view, the analyst and the analysand are both in a position of impossibility, with no common ground on which to stand together and separately, to create the inter-space which materialises the creative invitation to transference one of them makes to the other—the transferential offer of the analyst which precedes and conditions the analysand's transference.

* * *

Let us start at the end, in every sense of the word. The date is 2 October 1932, a few months before Ferenczi's death, and the text is a quotation from the end of his *Clinical Diary*:

> Further regression to being dead. (Not yet being born is the danger …)
>
>   In my case the blood-crisis arose when I realized that not only can I not rely on the protection of a "higher power" but *on the contrary* I shall be trampled under foot by this indifferent power as soon as I go my own way and not his …
>
>   Scientific achievements, marriage, battles with formidable colleagues—all this was possible only under the protection of the idea that *in all circumstances* I can count on the father-surrogate. Are the "identification" with the higher power, the most *sudden* "formation of the superego" the support that once preserved me from final disintegration? Is the only possibility for my continued existence the renunciation of the largest part of one's own self, in order to carry out the will of that higher power to the end (as though it were my own)?
>
>   And now, just as I must build new red corpuscles, must I (if I can) create a new basis for my personality, if I have to abandon as false and untrustworthy the one I have had up to now? Is the choice here one between dying and "rearranging myself"—and this at the age of fifty-nine?[9]

Everything has been said in a few words, and first of all the unwelcome transference, the rejected address to Freud, the original disappointment of a refusal to be acknowledged, and its repetition by Freud. The theory of mutual analysis can be seen as a manifestation of a request for an analysis *for* Freud, so that he might become an analyst, instead of remaining merely the self-analyst who invented psychoanalysis. In addition, we must take into account the limitations of the patient's self-analysis, undertaken to compensate for the faulty psychic presence of the analyst to himself, a deficiency which condemns the patient to a kind of paradoxical solitude: a solitude accompanied by the *deficient* psychic presence of the other, repeated or re-experienced with the analyst, which forces the subject to effect a deathly incorporation of this deficiency in himself—that is, to disappear *for* himself and *to* himself.

Of course, we must remember that the death drive is defined as a natural leaning towards self-annihilation, a leaning Freud described in *Civilisation and Its Discontents*, but with an open question beyond Freud, concerning self-destructiveness rooted in the incorporation of the self-destructiveness of the other. Finally, before discussing the traumatic experience, we must present a theory of the place (or rather, no place) of the trauma, as a split between affective regression and greater understanding, combining the endless disappearance of a part of oneself and end-less self-observation—in other words, the close interrelation between bleeding out in a dash towards death (that can be psychical or somatic) and the creative excite-ment of the thinking process, with no possible relief.

Everything has been said: it has been said with the urgency of a testament in the *Clinical Diary*, which records the destructiveness and the creativity ensuing from the request for analysis made to Freud.

The "analytic relation" between Ferenczi and Freud encounters obstacles, since it is inscribed in a passionate friendship that was to become stormy. For Ferenczi, it was obvious that their mutual transferences had to be worked through: this illusory obsession never left him. The mutual working through never really took place; it would have required the action of a third factor, which they partially and tempo-rarily found through cooperative scientific creativity, after the three segments of analysis, for about 12 years, which came to an end in the manner we all know. In other words, the analytic relation shifted place, moving beyond their personal rela-tion, into a space that offered no reliable and viable commonly constructed ground or thirdness: inevitably, a place condemned to disappear, the place where psychoa-nalysis was to start over. This new beginning was initiated by Ferenczi with and against Freud, *but never without him*.

The origin of the analyst's hindrance—and therefore of that which affects analysis—is double. It is related to Freud's inability to acknowledge and treat the negative aspect of Ferenczi's transference—this Freud who compensates for not being analysed by undertaking the self-analysis which sustains the creative process of psychoanalysis. Ferenczi is condemned to find an analyst for Freud in the new start he gives psychoanalysis with and against Freud, with and against himself. But this new start has a murderous component, given that their respective transferences intersect, annulling the possibility of a symbolic and symbol-generating matricide by means of the phantasmatic murder of the mother in Freud—the possibility of consenting to let her go without carrying out the murder on oneself.

Killing the mother in Freud: on one side, there is the supposedly unconditional love of Freud's mother and the "golden" son's maternal investment which protects him from disidealisation of the father and from fraternal rivalry; on the other side, there is the supposedly unconditional lack of love of Ferenczi's mother, transferred onto Freud by a son accused of his mother of killing her, and thus a son exposed to idealisation of the father and to fraternal rivalry.

This double hindrance—to Freud in being Ferenczi's analyst and to Ferenczi in being Freud's analysand—explains the *mutual* inability to turn murder into a phantasmatic scene, and make self-destructive action unnecessary. Together and incompletely separated, they inflict self-destructive behaviour on their relation-ship, and therefore on the creative power of the psychoanalysis *between them*. After them, the responsibility for what happened between them falls on every analyst, who must begin psychoanalysis anew on Freud's foundations and then follow in Ferenczi's footsteps, but differently: in the service of creativity rather than destructiveness.

Each analyst must re-enact the new start that Ferenczi introduced from an unprecedented place, and it is legitimate that those who follow do not expect to pay the same price, if they set aside the obligation to fill the analyst's place for their own analysts—*imaginarily* concentrated in a presumably undifferentiated transferential figure which they will have to learn to deconstruct in order to identify its components: the identificatory sources of his transference. Here, differentiating between transferential assignments waiting to be analysed is essential, to lighten the load upon the analyst of what was left unanalysed in his analysts, and to render bearable the confrontation with the inevitable limits of the analysable, which evolve and vary from one person to another.

* * *

Ferenczi's critics and proponents alike agree that Ferenczi's theory of transference is inseparable from his theory of trauma, as the text on confusion of tongues makes very clear. This text, Ferenczi's last, was the one Freud found almost impossible to accept, and this rejection is still, no doubt, at the heart of a controversial attitude toward Ferenczi.

Regardless of the nature of the traumatic experience, its seriousness and its early occurrence, the patient must be able to make the analyst a "witness" to a past event left unrepresentable until then. To achieve this, the analyst must play his role in the transference as a "well-meaning and helpful observer," because he becomes "the only possible witness" to the traumatic experience.[10] In order to become representable, the traumatic past must be brought into the present in the transference. The degree and quality of "being convincing" that this presentation/representation achieves, presuming the analyst plays his testimonial role, will determine the therapeutic action. In this process, the conception of transference is different than Freud's.

While Freud emphasises the elaborative offer of interpretation, considering it the final goal of transference, Ferenczi considers transference the vector of affects brought into the present. The interpretation of reminiscences is no longer what leads to the creative construction/reconstruction of the past; rather, repetition in the transference becomes the object of interpretation, through the patient's relived affective experiences, presented and brought into the present by their transferential function. Thus, working through involves the transformation of repeated elements into usable memories.

Ferenczi's approach to countertransference, based on the concept of tact, is very useful here. To understand this concept, we must return to the question of self-analysis. We know that Freud created psychoanalysis through a process of self-analysis to which he was constrained by his patients' experience of transference. Nevertheless, in the construction of Freud's edifice this self-analysis precedes and determines the *theorisation* of transference, which only emerges in the aftermath of the Dora case. When Ferenczi requested that Freud analyse him, he encountered the *self-analyst*: Freud, the self-analyst who invents psychoanalysis and proclaims himself a psychoanalyst. In other words, a negative figure of the relation between them, an intermediary figure, perhaps a hybrid, between them: between each one's resistance to the negativity of the transference and to the solitude it implies.

But just as Freud's self-analysis was unprecedented and impossible to repeat, because it created psychoanalysis, Ferenczi's self-analysis was unprecedented and impossible to repeat because it addressed Freud in a double manner from the start, as analyst *and* as the creator of psychoanalysis. Of course, in both cases, the predominant support of self-analysis is writing to another—mainly the *Correspondence*. Strictly speaking, self-analysis, that is, the self-analytic process, can only be put in writing by a third party after the interpretation of its reconstitution based on its written traces. Still, the letters exchanged by Freud and Ferenczi differ from those Freud exchanged with Fliess, on one fundamental point: when Ferenczi sent Freud the written account of his self-analysis, he presumed both Freud the analyst *and* the corpus he created to be *already present*. The main objective of Ferenczi's written self-analysis was to induce Freud to fill his role as analyst, to render him present and representable as an analyst.

This is the most obvious intention of the 26 December 1912 letter to Freud, which ushers in the three sequences of analysis conducted between 1914 and 1916. This letter should be read keeping in mind transferential ramifications related to Ferenczi's complicated relation with Gizella,[11] and to the consequences of Freud's personal involvement in that relation. This letter also refers back to the inaugural character of the Palermo conflict in September 1910, when Freud, who was working on the concept of paranoia, asked Ferenczi to act as his secretary, while Ferenczi expected to be his collaborator and contribute his own ideas. This dispute would later constitute a covert motive for Ferenczi's self-analysis and for his three sequences of analysis with Freud. At the end of these sequences, the situation was reversed when Freud asked Ferenczi to collaborate with him on a project on Lamarckism, with the express intention of diverting him from his wish to take up the analysis again.[12]

The content of Freud's 26 October 1916 letter mentioned earlier is ambiguous. In it, Freud plays with the distinction between "finished" and "terminated" analysis, which was to gain great interest within the psychoanalytic movement, as we know: "When I said the treatment was at an end, I did not mean it was terminated." The two men's collaboration on the Lamarck project was never realised—it took over a year for them to admit that it never would—and this failure demonstrated that it was impossible for them to invent psychoanalysis together, a desire signalled by Ferenczi's request for analysis. This impossibility was displaced, manifesting itself in Freud's inability to be Ferenczi's analyst, and in Ferenczi's inability to be Freud's analysand. Their reciprocal resistances reveal the function of mutual analysis for Ferenczi, the analyst: an attempt to explain his ambivalence towards Freud, infallible master and fallible analyst, because he lacks the personal experience of undergoing analysis with another analyst.

This ambivalence is also visible in his ambivalence towards his self-analysis, in which he also analyses Freud; self-analysis cannot replace analysis, and Ferenczi feels that this fact, obvious to him, *should* also be so to Freud—although this is not the case. On 2 September 1914, just before the first sequence of analysis, Ferenczi wrote Freud:

> The newest escape that should lead me out of this monotony is an attempt at self-analysis. The idea, to be sure, came to me only today; but I notice that I could still at least begin this work … But I have on no account totally given up the other idea (to be analyzed by *you*).[13]

Before, during and after the three segments of analysis—differently each time— Ferenczi's discussion of his self-analysis stays in the context of a transferential address to Freud as analyst, or more specifically, as an analyst unable to consent to the position of analyst. *Before*, there was the 26 December 1912 letter, followed by the one I just quoted: the self-analytic work can naturally be supposed to lead to a request for analysis. *During* the treatment, self-analysis is a way to continue the analytic work, despite its interruptions, in letters addressed to Freud. On 27 October 1914, just after the first interruption, Ferenczi wrote:

> I will … have to conduct our correspondence, at least in part, on an analytical basis. The sudden breaking off of our doctor-patient relationship (you see, I am writing as if in free association) would otherwise be all too painful for me. In addition, difficult to carry out … I spent my first free afternoon (the day before yesterday) conducting self-analysis in writing. It went smoothly; I imagined I was talking to you.[14]

After: The self-analytic writing addressed to Freud was intended to process the relinquishment of Freud as analyst. But Ferenczi seems aware of the impasse in which he finds himself when he continues to address himself to Freud in order to work through psychoanalytically his willingness to give him up as his analyst. This is clear in the letter dated 28 and 29 November 1916, shortly after the end of the third segment of analysis:

> I must also concede that I haven't achieved anything with the self-analysis. Possibly I really confused the situation. So, I will give it up. At the same time I also want thereby to free myself from your influence on my decisions—in the way that I made myself independent of Gizella through the separation. So, in these weeks I will write little …

And he cannot help adding a post-scriptum:

> P.S. I know only too well that it is in here a matter of the repetition of the defiant rebellion in Palermo—I already knew this while I was writing the letter—but I didn't want to withhold these characteristic associations from you.[15]

The impasse is made more serious by the fact that putting an end to self-analysis had been advised—not to say prescribed—by Freud, because of the risk of prolonging the transference on him indefinitely; just as not going through with marrying Gizella had also been advised by him. What could resolve this cruel paradox?

* * *

Ferenczi would try to do what Freud did: associate self-analysis with the creative process of psychoanalytic theory—but in his case, he could only start it over, not begin it. Unable to attribute self-analysis to the creative process, Ferenczi remained preoccupied with his transference to Freud. This transference is particular, mixed with envious hatred for Freud, not as an exceptional analyst, but rather as a *unique* self-analyst: the only *self-psychoanalyst*. That is, the only psychoanalyst who can enact a self-engendering fantasy, can attain self-realisation as the self-sufficient subject of a creation whose origins and foundation depend absolutely and exclusively on his subjective conceptual sphere. Freud, the self-psychoanalyst, is still the only one who can claim to be the only legitimate depositary of the *controlled designation* of a conceptual work brought forth by his psyche. The fact remains that this work is destined to be transmitted to others and enhanced by them—potentially, by all future psychoanalysts, *provided they invest it as their common origin*—as a fantasmatic scene presumably uniting Freud with each analyst, in a claim (avowed or denied) of exclusivity.

Ferenczi was hopelessly eaten up with (drowning in?) this envious transference which, by its very nature, could not be adequately worked through. This transference could only be addressed to Freud, and Freud couldn't help refusing to receive it, absorbed as he was in his transference to psychoanalysis. Freud's transference compensated for his inadequacy as Ferenczi's analyst, on condition that the transferential elements not be interpreted by any analyst, *starting with Ferenczi*. As a way out of this dilemma, the latter tried to reproduce the Freudian transference on psychoanalysis by transferring his disappointment in an analyst on the self-analytic work related to the construction of a theoretical edifice; to accomplish this, a connection had to be established between trauma and transference.

But this could not be done, since it also meant finding a theory offering an interpretation of Freud as a deficient analyst, given his lack of experience as an analysand. Not only is this unacceptable to Freud, but above all, such a theory can only be formulated from the position of a murderous child who does away with Freud's identification to his work and by his work. In other words, Ferenczi is irrevocably forced to construct a theory of psychoanalysis which is a deadly threat to him and to Freud, to each of them and to both of them together. Indeed, Ferenczi's reflection always threatened to remain focused on that which Freud lacked as his analyst: as if thinking served no purpose other than compensation.

No doubt, Ferenczi knew he was right about something essential. And no doubt, psychoanalysts must learn to carry on his legacy where this point is concerned.

That is, when the practice requires that, *with some patients*, the analyst accept to be confronted with the transferential repetition of a traumatic climate related to the psychic absence of the other, the one primordial for the *infans*, that is, related to a failure of incarnation of the *Nebenmensch*. It was not until early 1930 that Ferenczi was able to assume his own research fully, with Freud's knowledge, although it involved the latter's failure as an analyst:

> Now, in the relationship between you and me, it is (at least in me) a matter of the most diverse conflicts of feeling and attitude. First you were my revered teacher and unattainable model, for whom I harbored the, as you well know, not completely unalloyed feelings of an apprentice. Then you became my analyst, but the unfavorable conditions did not permit carrying out my analysis to completion. I was especially sorry that you did not comprehend and bring to abreaction in the analysis the partly only transferred, negative feelings and fantasies. As is well known, no analysand can do that without help ... Painstaking self-analysis was therefore required, which I consequently undertook and carried out quite methodically. Naturally this was also linked to the fact that I was able to abandon my somewhat puerile attitude and realize that I must not depend quite so *completely* on your favor.

And he adds a little further in the same letter:

> I do not, e.g. share your view that the process of healing is an unimportant procedure, or one that should be neglected ... only because it doesn't appear to us to be so interesting.[16]

This clearly shows how painful it was for Ferenczi to abandon his dependency on Freud. It was wrenching to be disappointed in him, while perceiving himself as disappointing. Not unlike what happens in a context of melancholia ...

Indeed, Ferenczi refers to their different points of view on melancholia, as they were expressed in their discussions on the subject of Freud's text "Mourning and Melancholia." For instance, on 25 February 1915, Ferenczi wrote:

> What you call a *projection* of the object shadow onto the narcissistic ego, I would rather call *intro*jection ... The occasion for the illness was effected by the disappointment in other persons who served as models for the narcissistic ego and the devaluation of whom also reveals one's own worthlessness. Melancholia is thus a case of unfortunate (unworthy) falling in love with one's self ...[17]

How can one love oneself if one was not loved by the primordial other at the stage of complete dependence? That is, without having experienced the other's ability to make one able to love himself? Ferenczi's reflection focused from the start on the origin of disappointment, a subject which, years later, would lead to the theory formulated in "The Unwelcome Child and His Death-Instinct." The personal question of his own transference is not separate from Ferenczi's understanding of transference as a possible repetition of the other's deficient psychic presence, at the root of the *infant's own disappointing-being* impression—since he introjected/incorporated the disappointment of the primordial other.

Ferenczi paid a heavy price for attempting to bring together technique and metapsychology, his remodelling of the Freudian concept of transference—as regards transference hatred and countertransference—and a new trauma theory. Here, it is important to point out the inherent connection between the 1928 paper "The Elasticity of Psycho-Analytic Technique" and the metapsychological reworking proposed in 1929 in "The Unwelcome Child."[18]

The figure of the wise baby should also be re-examined, that is, the figure representing the one who knows what he cannot know, and thus becomes the very representation of the limits of self-analysis. In any case, the 1928 text asserts that, for the analyst, self-analysis is necessary but not sufficient in order to process the patient's transference successfully: what is needed is constant oscillation between "empathy and self-observation" before forming "an opinion." This requires reserve on the analyst's part, in conveying his interpretations:

> Above all, one must be sparing with interpretations, for one of the most important rules of analysis is to do no unnecessary talking; over-keenness in making interpretations is one of the infantile diseases of the analyst. When the patient's resistance has been analytically resolved, stages in the analysis are reached every now and then in which the patient does the work of interpretation practically unaided, or with only slight prompting from the analyst.[19]

The same year, Ferenczi expounded on this idea at a conference given in Madrid, on the training of the analyst. Self-analysis can only partly overcome resistances, while those of a patient in analysis can be overcome completely, provided the analyst shows himself capable of tact. Acquiring tact presupposes having undergone analysis and having been involved in supervision, which Ferenczi described as a kind of "apprenticeship."[20]

***

I will not attempt to discuss here Ferenczi's different technical propositions which, through a continuous process of self-criticism, lead to mutual analysis. I only wish to examine the meaning of this outcome in light of what he wrote to Freud on 14 February 1930:

> I would only like to contradict you on one point: analytically open talking things out on no account means, in my view, that I am pressing you back into the role of the analyst and in so doing am relinquishing that of the tried-and-true friend.

My, I think, not unjustified hope extends to the point where an analytically free talking things out can be possible, even between old friends. I must admit that I would no longer feel good in the one-sided role of the analysand. Do you consider such mutual openness impossible?[21]

The idea of mutual analysis signals Ferenczi's willingness to give up the hope of being Freud's analysand, as well as any remaining notion of offering to be his analyst. Even more than he did in the case of the active technique or the question of elasticity, in the case of mutual analysis he focuses his theorising on his own psychic functioning in the session. Here we must refer to Elisabeth Severn, Ferenczi's patient and pupil who, in the *Clinical Diary*, plays a central role in considerations related to the "limits of application" of this technique.[22] Ferenczi's aim is to develop a theory concerning the conditions necessary to think through the countertransference.

On 3 June 1932,[23] when he asserts that mutual analysis is only a stop-gap measure compared to real analysis, he is protesting against didactic analysis and, at the same time, pointing out the limits of supervision. An analyst whose analysis was thorough enough can increase his ability for self-observation and judgement in the session, can place empathy and frustration in a dialectical relation[24] within the transferential context, and thereby have better control of his countertransferential actions, including in the interpretive work and in the imparting of his interpretations.

In the *Clinical Diary*, Ferenczi answers the insistent question of how far mutual analysis should be taken by saying: far enough for the patient to trust the possibility of being listened to, which will take the place of the infant's initial traumatic solitude, that seeks to repeat itself in the adult patient's transference. Beyond the traumatising event itself, the *wounded and misunderstood infans* evokes, for Ferenczi, the solitude inflicted by the faulty psychical presence to oneself and therefore to others of the primordial other on whom the *infans* depended for his survival.

The analyst's listening, which tactfully balances empathy and frustration, is required to help the patient bear the "pain of analytic weaning" and reinforce his ability to experience non-traumatic solitude, even though this may be at the limit of his possibilities: a situation where "he can only count on himself,"[25] Being able to experience solitude in this manner presupposes "sympathy" for the *infans* in the adult,[26] that is, sympathy for the internal alterity of the other as a different fellow human being. Here, sympathy does not refer to empathy for the analysand, but rather to an empathic enough investigation of his psychic functioning, which helps him to bear the frustration associated with being alone in the presence of the other, to use Winnicott's terminology.

It is with respect to these processes, beyond considerations related to mutual analysis, that Ferenczi opened and developed a perspective which continues to shed light on the psychic functioning of the analyst in the session.

Before considering Piera Aulagnier's "free-floating theorisation," and Winnicott's theory on countertransference, this perspective formed the basis of my notions of "internal witness" or "internal interlocution": something like an "internal mutuality" created by the words of the internal discourse, more than the internal supervision Anglo-Saxon descriptions often allude to. What is being described is how the analyst in the session talks to himself while listening to his listening; in other words, how the analyst observes himself, through the words that come to his mind, in the investigation of his psyche affected by the patient's transference.

The aim of this internal dialogue in context is, also, to find a way of "half-saying," between thinking and repression, in situations where the patient's transferential identifications intersect with the analyst's transference. Thus, the analyst develops his countertransference and invests it, at the same time, as a protective shield.[27] In other words, he introduces the thinkable where harmful experiences of the patient's archaic past and of his own unanalysed past could provoke countertransferential, interpretive or other behaviour—especially at the level of narcissistic identifications, electively adopted by borderline patients.

Ferenczi concluded that there was only one solution to such collusions, and he was the first to theorise it: namely, that the analyst be constantly aware of his own psychic functioning, and of how he uses psychoanalysis as a body of knowledge.[28] This requires that he examine his own unanalysed transferential traces, far enough back to uncover what was left unanalysed in his analysts. This is the role internal interlocution plays in the session. In its aftermath, this interlocution can—particularly when combined with writing, but not exclusively—provide the material and context needed to enable theoretical elaboration, that is, to serve the purposes of research into means of renewing psychoanalysis based on the unprecedented in each analysis, be it only by stimulating reflection among analysts in an effort to render the experience of transference shareable. As Winnicott has expressed it best:

> Psycho-analytic research is perhaps always to some extent an attempt on the part of the analyst to carry the work of his own analysis further than the point to which his own analyst could get him.[29]

The patient makes the analyst think with his affects and his body, that is, by affecting the analyst's thinking, sometimes to the point of making him uneasy. More than this: the analyst's thinking stems from the analysand's thinking, to such an extent that an author like Daniel Widlöcher has suggested the notion of "co-thinking" to underscore the fact that the analyst's associations *portray* the analysand's psychic reality.[30] This means that every interpretation carries within it a self-investigation supported by internal interlocution, which creates an internal space of thirdness, a space of self-investigation prompted by the search for the truth. Thus, the analyst's self-investigation, which aims at making possible that of the patient, requires the former to look into his past experiences as an analysand. This investigation may include questioning the ways of thinking and acting of his analysts, through their effects on him and on the transferential availability he offers his analysands—but without succumbing to the temptation of acting as his analyst's analyst in the transference onto his patient, which is perhaps what lies at the heart of all countertransferential action.

***

The fact that Ferenczi's thought was only granted its rightful place with difficulty and after much delay is no doubt due to a lack of understanding of his foundational role *and* the role of the questions raised by his clinical experiments. But, above all, what had to be avoided was the unbearable necessity of acknowledging the murderous potential of psychoanalysis at its inception, once we admit that it was not invented by Freud alone. This task is only unbearable for analysts because it reveals another task, which is hidden. Analysts must still accept that in their thinking process[31] the primordial difficulty lies in transforming their experience as analysands into a source of creativity. The task is to draw on this past experience as it exists in the present situation, as it is enacted in the present interaction of the hybrid elements of the transference, which carry the traces of the unanalysed transferences of their own analysts …

In truth, what we are dealing with is not Freud and Ferenczi's failure, but rather the sanctioning in and for oneself, of the coexistence of the analyst and the analysand, during the infinite number of their interactions, at all levels, from affects to thoughts.

Each psychoanalyst has to authorise the resolution of the Freud–Ferenczi dialogue, and deploy its creative power, rather than its destructive potential. Granting this authorisation requires solid grounding in the inexpressible solitude sharable between psychoanalysts—a solitude constituting the foundation of the symbolic community of analysts, irrespective of particular affiliations. The prerequisite for this authorisation is acceptance by the analyst of the limits of the analysable, and his willingness to forgo acting as his analysts' analyst—including being Freud's analyst: forgo identifying with the analyst Freud could not have or be, for himself and for Ferenczi. The one requirement left is to persist in *imagining* one's own analysts in the analytic situation, in the role of analyst *and* analysand.

Notes

1 This chapter reproduces the text of a conference given before the Quatrième Groupe on 6 October 2018 in Paris. Previously published in *Le Coq-Héron*, 239, 2019 (*Penser avec Ferenczi les pensées de l'analyste*).

2 Ferenczi, S., "The Elasticity of Psychoanalytic Technique," in *Further Contributions to the Theory and Practice of Psycho-Analysis*, Routledge, 1994 [1928].

3 Ferenczi, S., "The Elasticity of Psychoanalytic Technique," in *Further Contributions to the Theory and Practice of Psycho-Analysis*, Routledge, 1994 [1928].

4 Faldezer, E. and Brabant, E. (Eds.), *The Correspondence of Sigmund Freud and Sandor Ferenczi, 1914–1919*, Vol. 2, Harvard University Press, 1993.

5 A creative self-analysis: of psychoanalysis and of the first psychoanalyst.

6 Lugrin, Y., *Ferenczi on Freud's Couch: A Finished Analysis?* Routledge, 2021.

7 Faldezer, E. and Brabant, E. (Eds.), *The Correspondence of Sigmund Freud and Sandor Ferenczi, 1914–1919*, Vol. 2, Harvard University Press, 1993.

8 This is the perspective presented by Yves Lugrin in Lugrin, Y., *Ferenczi on Freud's Couch: A Finished Analysis?* Routledge, 2021.

9 Ferenczi, S., *The Clinical Diary of Sandor Ferenczi*, Harvard University Press, 1988.

10 Ferenczi, S., *The Clinical Diary of Sandor Ferenczi*, Harvard University Press, 1988.

11 This relation goes well beyond Ferenczi's romantic hesitation between Gizella and her daughter Elma, who was his patient for a time.

12 Yves Lugrin's reconstitution of all these events is entirely convincing, although I differ with his conclusion, which is to consider this 26 December 1912 letter a "first session." Lugrin, Y., *Ferenczi on Freud's Couch: A Finished Analysis?* Routledge, 2021.

13 Faldezer, E. and Brabant, E. (Eds.), *The Correspondence of Sigmund Freud and Sandor Ferenczi, 1914–1919*, Vol. 2, Harvard University Press, 1993.

14 Faldezer, E. and Brabant, E. (Eds.), *The Correspondence of Sigmund Freud and Sandor Ferenczi, 1914–1919*, Vol. 2, Harvard University Press, 1993.

15 Faldezer, E. and Brabant, E. (Eds.), *The Correspondence of Sigmund Freud and Sandor Ferenczi, 1914–1919*, Vol. 2, Harvard University Press, 1993.

16 Faldezer, E. and Brabant, E. (Eds.), *The Correspondence of Sigmund Freud and Sandor Ferenczi, 1914–1919*, Vol. 2, Harvard University Press, 1993, pp. 382–383.

17 Faldezer, E. and Brabant, E. (Eds.), *The Correspondence of Sigmund Freud and Sandor Ferenczi, 1914–1919*, Vol. 2, Harvard University Press, 1993.

18 Faldezer, E. and Brabant, E. (Eds.), *The Correspondence of Sigmund Freud and Sandor Ferenczi, 1914–1919*, Vol. 2, Harvard University Press, 1993.

19 Ferenczi, S., "The Elasticity of Psycho-Analytic Technique," in *Final Contributions to the Problems and Methods of Psycho-Analysis*, Routledge, 1994.

20 Ferenczi, S., "The Elasticity of Psycho-Analytic Technique," in *Final Contributions to the Problems and Methods of Psycho-Analysis*, Routledge, 1994.

21 Ferenczi, S., "The Training of the Analyst," Madrid Conference, 1928.

22 Faldezer, E. and Brabant, E. (Eds.), *The Correspondence of Sigmund Freud and Sandor Ferenczi, 1914–1919*, Vol. 2, Harvard University Press, 1993, p. 388.

23 Faldezer, E. and Brabant, E. (Eds.), *The Correspondence of Sigmund Freud and Sandor Ferenczi, 1914–1919*, Vol. 2, Harvard University Press, 1993, p. 388.

24 Faldezer, E. and Brabant, E. (Eds.), *The Correspondence of Sigmund Freud and Sandor Ferenczi, 1914–1919*, Vol. 2, Harvard University Press, 1993, p. 388.

25 Faldezer, E. and Brabant, E. (Eds.), *The Correspondence of Sigmund Freud and Sandor Ferenczi, 1914–1919*, Vol. 2, Harvard University Press, 1993, p. 388.

26 Faldezer, E. and Brabant, E. (Eds.), *The Correspondence of Sigmund Freud and Sandor Ferenczi, 1914–1919*, Vol. 2, Harvard University Press, 1993, p. 388.

27 This question was fully theorised by Pierre Fédida. See Fédida, P., *Crise et contre-transfert*, PUF, 1992, p. 170.

28 See Fédida, P., *Crise et contre-transfert*, PUF, 1992, p. 170.

29 Winnicott, D., "Hate in the Counter-Transference," *Journal of Psychotherapy Practice and Research*, 3 (4), 1994 [1947].

30 See Widlöcher, D., "Empathy and Co-Thinking," *Journal de la Psychanalyse de l'Enfant*, 3 (2), 2013: 39–44.

31 As it applies to the treatment process, and inspired by the experience of transference, whether thinking from the perspective of an analysis, that of any other "analytic" structure, or that of a non-clinical context.

Chapter 4

Beginning, Starting Over[1]

The Ferenczian renewal does not consist simply of reconsidering the dialectics of the beginnings and new beginnings of psychoanalysis. Based on clinical practice, and on borderline psychopathology, this renewal requires reconsideration of the question of the frame, and more generally the conditions needed to shed light on the gaps between site, situation and process. Indeed, so-called borderline patients bring into question very directly certain constitutive gaps between the frame and the analyst who provides the frame, between the person of the analyst and the object of the transference, between (interpretive and self-interpretive) listening and interpretation (communicated or not).[2]

* * *

The borderlines sphere tends to oblige the analyst to adapt *endlessly* to the different forms of the transferential demand, until the mode of identification produced corresponds most closely to the analysand's transferential needs. The borderline patient seeks to bring about a shared belief in a concordance of the past and the present, in a relation of coincidence between himself and his transference, and between the analyst and the object of the transference. The transferential material is confused, showing a state of archaic despair, mixing identification with the terrorised child, and with the narcissistic mother, as if the adult carried inside him the *infans* once confronted with a deficient mother-environment.

In my view, this borderline picture results from the unrepresentable despair associated with the Ferenczian unwelcome child, a despair reactivated in the transference in the form of a disappointment appearing to be reciprocal. In borderline transference, the analyst is expected to experience and to inflict disappointment, or to be disappointed/disappointing, because his psychic presence is unbearable for the patient and must be attacked, since it contains an unthinkable promise and reveals the appeal to the other, contained in his request.

The attack takes the form of a murderous action through words: to eliminate the experience of being heard, in the listening granted by the other. The request to be heard is denied or negated in a discourse reduced to the recitation of countless

DOI: 10.4324/9781003542483-6

unfounded reasons for disappointment. The analyst is addressed in a manner intended to reduce him to an interlocutor without alterity, obliged to separate listening from speech: an interlocutor in the position of a spectator to a monologue staged as an impossible dialogue. What emerges is the paradoxical outline of a (possibly) therapeutic opening: desperate transference, without recognising itself as such, needs a witness.

For the patient, this witness is the third party to be attacked in person in the analyst, so as to *test* him, in order to *test* the one to whom the transference is addressed. This offers the analyst the possibility of filling the gap between the internal experience of the words and their transferential transmission through speech. All therapeutic results will depend on his manner of imagining this subjective experience of the patient, based on his own internal experience of words. What is crucial is the way in which he will work with the hybrid matter of his countertransferential affects, starting with an internal dialogue with the patient's words, so that they activate the multiple sources of words carried in his own transference, which includes transference on psychoanalysis: the creative expectation of unprecedented thoughts in the analysis.

The analyst's internal experience is the chosen target of the borderline patient; it is the psychic space in which he can locate his request, in the projective displacement of his experiences. He must evacuate the threatening precarity of his internal experience, contained in his words, by transforming it into the precarisation of that of the analyst. *The analyst's internal experience*: a sphere of words, of the analyst's listening to his listening and to what lies beyond it, in himself, and outside himself. In other words, the analyst's internal interlocution, the articulation in words of his internal alterity, testify, in and through their effects, to those of the analysand, which the latter tries to erase by erasing those of the other.

The challenge faced by the analyst in confronting the borderline sphere is to succeed in substituting absence for erasure. The analysand must erase himself as the actor of his erasure in the other, in order to recognise his own innocence and force the analyst to feel guilty for this erasure, to the point of self-hatred: hate of his inability to be there for the other. The analyst's feeling of guilt, not altogether unconscious, is an effect of borderline transference, but also a defensive strategy exerting a protective-shield and elaborative function.[3]

One of the reasons for choosing face-to-face therapy with borderline patients is that this situation allows the presence/absence of the analysts to be visible, reducing the risk of suicidal acting out related to this play centred on disappearance. The inevitable disadvantage is an additional technical difficulty, with a tendency to intensify interpretations, to fight against the confusion of psychical spaces, and to avoid intersubjective communication. Preserving the presentification of absence, despite the visibility of faces and postures, is made even more difficult by the defensive function of interpretations, too heavily laden with countertransferential reactions. This confirms Fédida's idea that psychotherapies are "complicated analyses" to be relegated to a "practice of difficult therapies," which remains to be defined.[4]

In a borderline context, everything depends on the analyst's presence to himself, in the silence of internal interlocution. Here, we would be well advised to consider the existence of an agency *instituting* the analyst's transference, an agency holding an intrinsic place in the analytic situation—an influence that the borderline sphere brings into question and, at the same time, makes most visible. Such a hypothesis would be in line with Michel Neyraut and André Green's works. Each of them has proposed a radical renewal of perspective by theorising the precedence of countertransference over transference, of the countertransferential offer over the transferential request. Neyraut went as far as asserting that countertransference is not only a response, but also constitutes a "demand."[5] However, as Jean-Paul Valabrega has clearly pointed out, the very idea of precedence must be set aside, since we cannot think of transference and countertransference in a relation of antecedence.[6]

It is not enough to consider that the patient's transference and the analyst's countertransference constitute one entity, or simply to grant affect all its importance in the countertransference, since it is clear that countertransferential affects are the source of interpretive work. Countertransference is not limited to an emotional reaction to the patient's transference, but involves the entire psychic functioning of the analyst in the session. From this point of view, countertransference cannot be considered separately from the impact of what we must call the analyst's transference. This requires taking into account continued developments since Freud, and the idea of countertransference as a limit. These developments, partly tied to considerations of the question of borderline, designate countertransference as a primordial factor determining the frame, and as the support of all interpretation.

***

Winnicott, the first theoretician of borderline psychology,[7] undoubtedly holds a central place in these developments, given his famous 1947 text, the best-known and most widely commented on.[8] His lesser-known, almost forgotten paper written 13 years later deserves some comment. "Countertransference" is a disconcerting text diverse and loosely structured, eluding easy play with Winnicottian terminology. Here, the perspective is no longer that of the wider 1947 conception of countertransference; on the contrary, this paper delegitimates that perspective. Winnicott asks: can countertransference be reduced to the analysand's interference with the analyst's manner of receiving the transference? He asks this question on the strength of his belief in the notion of a "professional attitude," allowing him to theorise the necessary gap between, on the one hand, the person of the analyst, and, on the other hand, the analyst as transferential object and guarantor of the therapeutic frame.

What the patient meets is surely the professional attitude of the analyst, not the unreliable, men and women we happen to be in private life[9] ... I would rather be remembered as maintaining that in between the patient and the analyst is the analyst's professional attitude, his technique, the work he does with his mind.[10]

In so far as all this is true the meaning of the word countertransference can only be the neurotic features *which spoil the professional attitude* and disturb the analytic process as determined by the patient.[11]

But in non-neurotic contexts, a professional attitude does not play the same role, be it with patients with antisocial tendencies or those with intense regressive needs.[12] As described in the 1954 article on regression,[13] patients in the latter category need to experience more or less total dependence in order to be in contact with their "true self," at the cost of salutary depression. Here, it is best that the analyst's professional attitude take a different form: the patient enters and then frees himself of transferential depression when he becomes "angry" about the analyst's past failures,[14] as Winnicott put it in his 1955 paper.

However, this transferential *present* can only become the past through countertransference: that is, as a *reaction* to transferential impact, more or less enacted, and generally repressed/denied; but also as a *response* requiring elaborative work. The analyst needs to be able to combine a professional attitude with creative tolerance of his own "vulnerability, which goes hand in hand with a flexible, defensive organisation."[15]

But this clinical and metapsychological advance founded—without specifying it—on the Ferenczian perspective with regard to metapsychology of the analyst's thought process in the session seems to be cancelled by the closing statement of the text, foretold from the beginning: "Would it not be better at this point to let the term countertransference revert to its meaning of that which we hope to eliminate by selection and analysis and the training of analysts?"[16]

This questionable ideal of eliminating countertransference through analysis and training serves the purpose of the idealisation of doing the work of elaborating the transference–countertransference dynamic. What this eliminates is the need for a metapsychological approach to countertransference, which borderline functioning requires. In truth, when Winnicott realised that he was making a promise he could not keep, he stepped back: he rejected a differential theory of countertransference that would take into account diagnostic, if not nosographic, criteria.

This text, with the unease and hesitations it displays, constitutes a concrete illustration of what was at stake in the debates about countertransference—discussions about a choice between a narrow or wide conception of it, which went so far as to question the legitimacy of the notion.

In this light, the text can serve as an incitement to think about what Winnicott overlooked: the idea that a part of the countertransference, or its acceptance, is not simply a reaction, or even a response to transference, but an offer made by the analyst, which precedes and influences the transference. This offer is particularly influential and visible in borderline functioning, which reveals the work of what we can only call the analyst's transference.

***

Thanks to Winnicott and a few others, today the analyst can consider himself "responsible for the transference, and accept this responsibility,"[17] as Patrick Guyomard beautifully expressed it in his reading of Lacan; he points out the latter's concept of analysis as an encounter of the patient's desire with the analyst's desire. Guyomard emphasises that although Lacan considers that the analyst's desire precedes the transference, he continues to use the term "countertransference."

Indeed, for Lacan, the aim is not to reject countertransference or this term, but rather to acknowledge the inadequacy of the term for rendering the transferential aspect of the analyst's involvement and his responsibility in the patient's transference. We would be well advised not to reduce countertransference to a reaction or an answer, but rather to see it as a means of attaining an internal positioning which makes it possible to bear a double responsibility:[18] for one's involvement in and through the patient's transference, and for the self-observation of this involvement, in the aftermath. It is here that the term "countertransference" proves to be insufficient, because this double responsibility is affected by the work related to the analyst's confrontation with the limits of his analysis and, above all, of his analysability: a responsibility to be accepted and used in his present work as a source of animation and as a convergence point in the elaboration of the countertransference.

Pierre Fédida makes it clear that the analyst must be able to imagine what the patient, as a fellow human being,[19] experiences. I would add that he must also continue to be able to imagine his own analyst(s) as analysts *and* as analysands, in a different way with each patient—which presupposes sufficient self-observation and self-questioning in his present situation as an analyst, and in the work of updating his past experiences as an analysand. In other words, the analyst's work of elaboration involves composing *evolving figures* of his analysts, in order to see himself work with identifications and counter-identifications, tied in with this work; but also to see himself work *differently*—specifically through the observation of his own resistances with his patients. Thus, the analyst's resistances follow the contours of the not yet analysed, waiting to become analysable, including in its resonance with the unanalysed in his analyst(s).

The desired aim is the taking into account of the plural and unstable character of the transferential material of the figurations of one's analyst: an evolving transferential composition, a changing mix always going beyond an individual's reality and beyond his way of being and acting in a particular situation. Alternating the singular with the plural is intended to emphasise that this transferential composition produces a figure of the interlocutor, albeit evolving and compounded: composed, as it were, of different faces, starting with but going beyond the analysts who trained the analyst—his analysts of reference, as we called them earlier.

From a Ferenczian point of view, we might say that borderline patients invite—even oblige or constrain—the analyst to continue his analysis, deepening an irremediable solitude related to the infinite nature of the internal encounter between the analysand and the analyst. Although it cannot be shared, this particular solitude is common to psychoanalysts as a necessarily peculiar personal experience felt, nevertheless, to be sharable—something that should prove to be true in supervisions (for both supervisor and supervised analyst), and in all situations bringing psychoanalysts together.

The borderline register imposes a confrontation between the analyst and the internalised fate of what remained unanalysed in his analysts; neurotic patients do no more than to invite such a confrontation. Patients in the borderline sphere, who must give up their invulnerability and be able to suffer[20]—and thus be able to identify with the analyst—need for the latter to experience his vulnerability and become aware of his repression, while maintaining a "professional attitude." I would redefine professional attitude as the analyst's disposition to be attentive to the enigma revived in him by the patient, concerning his largely unconscious identifications and counter-identifications to his analysts of reference. This attentiveness to the invisible is enacted in a particular manner: an internal interlocution that safeguards the "intimate stranger," the "site of the stranger,"[21] consisting of maintaining the gap between the subject who listens and the one to whom the speech is addressed.

The internal alterity at work in the analyst must be *maintained* for a dissymmetry between the analyst and the patient to be *maintained*—a dissymmetry the borderline patient claims to erase, in a perfectly incestuous manner, by using the analyst's limits *as* proof of the symmetry of their places. The borderline patient wants to legitimate the confusion between the analyst who interprets and the analyst *to be killed*, the target of transference hate and, therefore, the condition making possible an aim likely to make murder a reason for absence. The analyst confronted with the borderline register is faced with the question of how to avoid destroying the symbolic possibility of murder.

Following in the footsteps of Jean-Luc Donnet, Baldacci insists on "a function producing thirdness," when he equates the analyst's desire, as Lacan does, with "transference on analysis."[22] I see this as making reference to an original transference, the transference at the origins of psychoanalysis, founding a primal scene for the analyst and establishing his position: the intermediary position instituted by the *unliveable* dialogue, both destructive and creative, between Freud and Ferenczi.

***

... The reproduction of a new start between Freud and Ferenczi. The analyst's internal interlocution as I define it consists in part, for each analyst, of reiterating the founding dialogue at the start of psychoanalysis: with Freud imagining his future readers, called upon to be witnesses and interlocutors in a thinking process in progress. But in the renewal of psychoanalysis through the Freud-Ferenczi relation a resistance emerges—one that could be deadly to psychoanalysis—in the form of Ferenczi's analysis with Freud. Psychic murder—soul murder?—is committed *halfway*: by two people, Freud and Ferenczi, not targeting one or the other of them, but rather the psychoanalytic force of their dialogue.

One cannot be analysed by the other, but this impossibility, which leads to a passionate relationship, also reveals the creative and (self)destructive power of the polarity at work in psychoanalysis, of the duality at the heart of the process which created it. This creative duality, at first practised by Freud alone, continues in the form of a solitude for two: the transferential merger, unanalysable by nature, of the Freudian beginnings and the Ferenczian renewal. In other words, in hindsight, the original creative duality appears to have developed from the intersection of Freud's transference onto writing and the transferential renewal brought about by Ferenczi.

Some biographical facts are helpful here. On the one hand, Ferenczi, the child accused by his mother of killing her, and consequently torn between complicity with a murderous mother, against himself, and his fight to survive the internalisation of the accusation by turning the murder against the accuser. On the other hand, "*goldener Sigi*," finally enjoys his destiny of preferred son, while at the same time dreading his mother's death, not knowing if what he fears most is dying before her or the opposite. This is the situation as it exists concretely, with biographical or historical considerations remaining secondary.

As is the case for all analysts—given their unavoidable difference from Freud—for Ferenczi's theory has a self-theorising function which reaches its peak in the *Clinical Diary*. The "wise baby" and the "unwelcome child" are, of course, him! The fact that Ferenczi's work remained "unwelcome" for a long time, obstructed by the multiple, contradictory and passionate aims setting analysts against each other, is no doubt due to the difficulty of realising Ferenczi's founding role *and* the fundamental role of the questions raised by his clinical experiments. But the blame can also be placed, in large measure, on the unbearable task[23] of having to acknowledge the inaugural murderous component of psychoanalysis, once it became clear that it was not invented by Freud alone.

Attempted murder committed by Freud and Ferenczi against the creative force of their relation. It was not only that Freud could not respond to Ferenczi's *unwelcome* transferential need. Freud undoubtedly could not hear this need to address a murderous mother who accused her son of killing her. From his position as the creator and founder of psychoanalysis, Freud, who ultimately wanted to remain the only one entrusted with the transmission of his oeuvre, was condemned to condemn Ferenczi to being *unwelcome*.

This made Freud an unanalysable analyst, *excluded* from the position of analyst by the invention of psychoanalysis. Now, this *unwelcome* status is applied to an analysand—Ferenczi—who is himself unanalysable: in desperation, forced by his analyst without an analyst to try to compensate for the lack of an analyst by creating psychoanalysis. But psychoanalysis already existed, and the absence of an analyst for Freud is neither a fault nor a deprivation.

Indeed, while Freud compensated for not having an analyst by inventing psychoanalysis, Ferenczi could only attempt to reinvent it to compensate for Freud's inability to be his analyst. For Ferenczi, this inability, which Freud does not acknowledge, repeats the soul murder committed against her son by the mother who accused him of murder.[24] However, as the *Clinical Diary* testifies in retrospect, it is doubtless this impossible shared lack of an analyst that saves Ferenczi.

While this lack, which produced the temptation of being Freud's analyst in order to succeed in making him become his analyst at last, was catastrophic for Ferenczi, the shared lack of an analyst *saved him*. Or, at least, allowed him to partially transform murderous hatred into a source of creative thinking—the hatred being even more destructive by the impossibility of addressing it to anyone, since a subject for it could not be found.

Attempted murder against the Freud–Ferenczi relation, which would have lent its full force to the creative duality at the heart of Freud's creative process. We know that this attempt was facilitated, made official and, at the same time, hidden under cover of a psychiatric pseudo-diagnosis made by Ernest Jones regarding Ferenczi, more and more explicitly after 1927–1928. Jones, who had been analysed by Ferenczi, was seized with hate-filled envy aggravated by the feeling of *being excluded*—excluded from the initial Freud-Ferenczi complicity: he was neither a Jew, nor a friend, nor truly creative; and what's more, unlike them, he was an opponent of lay analysis. Something like the soul of psychoanalysis was at stake here.

From Freud's perspective, we could define the "soul" of psychoanalysis as that which animates it by animating each analyst; that is, there is a direct relation with the enigma of being and thinking, so that this enigma is used transferentially in the exploration of one's own psychic functioning, through and beyond one's analysts of reference. This examination is prompted by the tension between the surprising present relevance of the Freudian oeuvre, thanks to its successive renewals since Ferenczi, and the unprecedented singularity of each patient and each transferential demand. The soul of psychoanalysis can be thought to have emerged or appeared with the viewpoint produced by Freud's internal dialogue, which enabled him to invent psychoanalysis in a (self-)transferential process supported by writing.

For Freud, the creative process required thinking in the form of a dialogue, an internal scene of interlocution involving support from the reader taken as a witness and as an interlocutor, while his thinking was taking shape and proposing a genealogical perspective of its development. When addressing his readers, Freud always offers them a genealogy explaining the internal (and secondarily external!) sources of all new theoretical proposals. However, a problem remains: Freud needs to be surrounded by sympathetic persons who can embody this self-transferential material—sometimes at a great price to themselves. With the exception of Fliess, Ferenczi was the most strongly invested collaborator, and the most strongly resistant, given his own genius. But also given both men's ambivalence towards the child-therapist Ferenczi!

This point of view, at the same time a blind spot, produced by Freud's internal dialogue and passed on through his dialogue with Ferenczi, designates a virtual place to be recognised as such, and to remain virtual: the place of Freud's analyst. Analysts are constantly tempted to transform this place into a vacancy to be filled, given the narcissistic omnipotence they can't help attributing to their analysts and/ or to themselves. This is where we could consider the idea of a soul of psychoanalysis to be lodged: the enigma of the unknowable, to be discovered with each patient and made easier to live with for him, by means of the opening offered by his past for creating new possibilities for his future.

For this to happen, analysts must allow themselves to be *animated* by their internal dialogue, between the therapist and the researcher—a dialogue always likely to become conflictual, like it was for Freud, but in a different way, since it is located in an unforeseeable lineage: founded on filiation networks with indefinite connections. If the analyst refuses to be a researcher, he may cause more or less serious injury to the enigma at the heart of the psychic functioning of the patient: he may fail to turn the patient into a researcher who can recognise the traces of his affects in his own words and those of the analyst, provided he is sufficiently inspired by the transference.

The fact that the soul of psychoanalysis was dramatically mistreated by Jones when he succeeded in dislodging Ferenczi for decades from his place as Freud's chosen interlocutor should prompt psychoanalysts to prolong Freud's internal dialogue, by following in Ferenczi's footsteps, or in a different way. As a first step, analysts must allow the Freud–Ferenczi dialogue, with its conflicts, to continue and remain alive for each of them and among them. They must be able to analyse their past experiences as analysands through their present work in the analyses they conduct, to analyse unanalysed transferential remnants, as well as what is left of the transferences of their analysts, in the fixations that emerged in working with them. This requires more than just managing creatively the uncomfortable tension between what has already been conceived and what is still unthinkable. What is needed above all is to avoid being carried away by a phantasmatic vision, resistant and harmful if it becomes an imagined goal: becoming an analyst to analyse one's analysts of reference.

At the metapsychological level, Freud and Ferenczi both show us the original duality of psychoanalysis … *starting with* Freud in his solitary process of creation. They remind us that this creation is originally an initiation to the enigma of psychic life, where nothing is lost and everything potentially exists in the present. To the enigma of psychic life indissociably made up of an instinctual component and a cultural component, a narcissistic dimension and a sexual dimension, of a vital dependence register and an Oedipal register, a self-preserving aspect, and a self-destructive aspect …

Notes

1 This chapter and the next continue the work undertaken previously in various publications: "Cadre interne, transfert et contre-transfert," *Filigranes*, 2018; "Le contre-transfert de Winnicott: une chute qui donne à penser," *Le Coq-Héron*, 235, 2018; "Au commencement était le meurtre …" *Le Coq-Héron*, 224, 2016; "La crainte de l'effondrement," in Chagnon, J.-Y. (Ed.), *Commentaires de textes fondamentaux en psychopatologie psychanalytique*, Dunod, 2012, pp. 121–128.

2 In this context, we would do well to examine the beginnings of the therapy, and its variations, depending on whether it takes place in a private office or a treatment centre and weather in the centre in question an analyst receives the initial request for analysis, while another analyst conducts the sessions. I refer the reader to the distinction between the encounter and the first consultation, theorised by Jean-Luc Donnet, who asserts that the analytical aspect of the encounter always emerges only in the aftermath. This

dimension emerges after a process of assessment—a distinct process and, at the same time, a preliminary treatment—which leads to a decision: "excluding refusal" (Donnet, J.-L., *The Analyzing Situation*, Weller, A. (Trans.), Karnac, 2009).

3   Pierre Fédida has proposed a theory of "countertransference as a guilt-based strategy," "consisting of feeling guilty for the violence wrought by the other" (Fédida, P., *Crise et contre-transfert*, op. cit., p. 151).

4   Fédida, P., *Des bienfaits de la depression*, Odile Jacob, 2001, p. 159. See also Fédida, P., *Crise et contre-transfert*, PUF, 2009, p. 151.

5   Neyraut, M., *Le Transfert: étude psychanalytique*, PUF, 1976, p. 25.

6   Valabrega, J.-P., *La formation du psychanalyste*, Payot, 1994.

7   It bears repeating here, disconcerting as I have pointed out since 2011, that just as Winnicott is surely its first theoretician, Ferenczi is just as surely its pioneering, figure and founder, notwithstanding previous research, such as that of Helen Deutsch.

8   Winnicott, D., "Hate in the Countertransference,", *International Journal of Psycho-Analysis*, 30, 1949: 69–74.

9   Winnicott, D., "Counter-Transference," *Brit. J. Med. Psychol.*, 33, 1960: 17.

10 Winnicott, D., "Counter-Transference," *Brit. J. Med. Psychol.*, 33, 1960: 17.

11 Winnicott, D., "Counter-Transference," *Brit. J. Med. Psychol.*, 33, 1960: 17.

12 Winnicott, D., "Counter-Transference," *Brit. J. Med. Psychol.*, 33, 1960: 17.

13 Winnicott, D., "Metapsychological and Clinical Aspects of Regression within the Psycho-Analytical Setting," in *The Collected Works of D. W. Winnicott: Vol. 4, 1952–1955*, Caldwell, L. & Taylor Robinson, H. (Eds.), Oxford University Press, 2016 [1954].

14 Winnicott, D., "Clinical Varieties of Transference," in *Through Paediatrics to Psychoanalysis*, Routledge, 1975.

15 Winnicott, D., "Counter-Transference," *Brit. J. Med. Psychol.*, 33, 1960: 17.

16 Winnicott, D., "Counter-Transference," *Brit. J. Med. Psychol.*, 33, 1960: 17.

17 Guyomard, P., "Lacan et le contre-transfert: le contre-coup du transfert," in Guyomard, P. (Ed.), *Lacan et le contre-transfert*, PUF, 2011, p. 14.

18 The etymology of the word associates "to respond" with "to answer for."

19 Fédida, P., "Le psychanalyste: un état limite?," in André, J. and Thompson, C. (Eds.), *Transfert et états limites*, PUF, 2002, p. 92.

20 Winnicott, D., "The Concept of Clinical Depression Compared with that of Defence Organization," in *Collected Works*, Vol. 8, Oxford University Press, 2016 [1967].

21 Fédida, P., *Le site de l'étranger* (The Site of the Stranger), PUF, 2009.

22 Baldacci, J.-L., *L'analyse avec fin* (Analysing to an End), PUF, 2016.

23 An intolerable smear (in French, the words for "task" and "smear" are almost homonyms).

24 In the place where you need me to love you, I will not be and will not exist except through the displacement in you of my murderous hatred—a hatred denied by me and aroused by your need of me, a hatred you will have to take into yourself if you insist on living: so that, to stay alive, you will only be able to reach me by killing yourself, by dedicating yourself to (resisting) disappearance—yours, the other's.

Chapter 5

Welcoming the Unwelcome Child

The question of a second dualism arose inevitably between Freud and Ferenczi. "The Unwelcome Child and His Death-Instinct," which posits a tendency to self-destruction as a response to a destructive fault in the environment, draws us out of the sphere of strictly Freudian thought. We are asked to conceive of the death drive no longer through the prism of an approach based on individual constitution—a view clearly predominant in Freud's thinking—but rather from a perspective that allows for the particularities of a specific environment, although Ferenczi did not exclude the notion of a constitutional aspect of self-destruction.

The *Clinical Diary* is much more than the field of ruins of a dying man aware of his technical and metaphysical meanderings, and aware that Freud has deserted him. At the end of the *Clinical Diary*, it is clear that Ferenczi feels his death is near and strives to define the limits and problems associated with his search for technical innovations intended to bring an answer to the particularities of what we now call, for lack of a better term, borderline functioning.

This self-critical attitude reveals a passion for independent theorising, that no doubt reached its height and was more intense than ever in his relationship with Freud. But it is also the attitude needed to carry out the theoretical work of metapsychological reformulation, solidly rooted in clinical practice. Ferenczi confronted fully, in a creative and imaginative manner, the questions raised by the second drive theory, particularly the problem of the place of self-preservation, still pivotal today in discussions about the death drive.

Indeed, Ferenczi proposed another version of drive dualism, with two contradictory impulses: "drives for self-assertion" and "drives for conciliation."[1] Whether or not he tended to favour the idea of drive unicity shall be left for another discussion. What we wish to point out here is that his approach to drive dualism, which he described as an "apparently slight modification of the Freudian hypothesis of life and death pulses,"[2] leads to the idea of polarity (egoistic pole/altruistic pole.) This polarity restores the place of self-preservation through the egoistic pole, leading to cooperation of the drives in the service of life.

In this metapsychologically crucial text, Ferenczi focuses on externally caused self-destructiveness, rather than the internal tendency to self-destruction—too often

DOI: 10.4324/9781003542483-7

insufficiently distinguished from an instinct intrinsically oriented towards death—connected with repetition compulsion. By doing this, he casts doubt on the use of the Freudian term "death drive"; indeed, three years later, in the *Clinical Diary*, he would admit that he finds it hard to use this term.[3] Yet in 1929 he employed this term in the context of the metapsychological frame of the life and death instincts. Since the vital energy of the foetus, and then of the infant, is very limited, it is insufficient to protect him from a "tendency to self-destruction"; therefore, he cannot do without the parents' psychic protection and in case this protection is insufficient, the destructive impulses may take him back to the "individual non-being" which is still familiar to him.

> It is true that the organs and their functions develop at the beginning of life within and without the uterus with astonishing profusion and speed—but only under the particularly favourable conditions of germinal and infantile protective environment. The child has to be induced, by means of an immense expenditure of love, tenderness and care, to forgive his parents for having brought him into the world without any intention on his part; otherwise the destructive instincts begin to stir immediately. And this is not really surprising, since the infant is still much closer to individual non-being, and not divided from it by so much bitter experience as an adult. Slipping back into this non-being might therefore come much more easily to children. The "life-force" which rears itself against the difficulties of life has therefore not really any great innate strength, and becomes established only when tactful treatment and upbringing gradually give rise to progressive immunisation against physical and psychical injuries.[4]

Despite the coherent reasoning in the text, Ferenczi is unable to resolve a certain ambiguity about the concept of self-destruction. The foundations he lays connect it essentially to the external roots of a destructive fault in the environment,[5] while holding on to the idea of a "congenital" aspect of the "tendency to self-destruction." He seems unable to break completely with the Freudian position which, for all intents and purposes, ignores the effects of the environment on the construction of the infant's psyche, and which extends the death drives beyond destructive instincts. Indeed, it is quite clear that Ferenczi sees the death drives essentially as instincts of self-destruction, neglecting the Freudian idea of the tendency to reduce tension and to return to an inorganic state.

* * *

The child has to be induced, by means of an immense expenditure of love, tenderness and care, to forgive his parents for having brought him into the world without any intention on his part; otherwise the destructive instincts begin to stir immediately.

The external sources of self-destruction do not consist simply of an inadequate maternal holding or shielding function. What is involved relates to narcissism, and solving the problem requires a theory of narcissism—different than Freud's 1914 theory—which can take into account the role of the environment. After introducing the death drive, Freud does not return to the question of narcissism—although the introduction of narcissism announces the death drive; Ferenczi questions Freud's death drive theory, but does not go as far as questioning narcissism. This would be left to Winnicott.

Winnicott's metapsychological model of the maternal face/gaze as an identifying mirror would shed light on the necessity for the convergence of the infant's narcissistic and objectal investments, if he is held and contained well enough, and if the object is presented to him well enough. Later, André Green's work was to provide a reformulation bringing together narcissism and death instinct.[6] Green was a self-proclaimed disciple of Winnicott, who was himself tacitly a disciple of Ferenczi: a "Winnicottian" psychoanalyst who went beyond Winnicott's rejection of the death drive, by recentering the second drive dualism on the polarity life instinct/destruction instinct.

It is commonly accepted in the analytic milieu that Freud's weakness consists in his mistaken theorisation of the role of the "object" in mental development; moreover, the term "object" is inherently problematic. Green rightly objects to the contemporary opposition made between drive theory and object relations theory, since this opposition maintains Freud's underestimation of the role of the object. Green also reminds us very fittingly that, since the function of the object is to facilitate the intrication of the libido with destructiveness, we cannot altogether exclude the possibility that many disintrications are related to the consequences of the response to the object.[7]

Because for Green the psychopathology of limits is a primary consideration, he grants a central role to the concept of a destructive drive and emphasises the possible disintrication of Thanatos and Eros, while objecting to approaches that tend to reduce Eros to connection and Thanatos to disconnection. Eros and Thanatos both include connection and intrication, as well as disconnection and disintrication, but the first pair is predominant with Eros and the second with Thanatos. This makes it possible to identify self-destruction characteristic of borderline pathologies—especially thoughts of self-mutilation entirely beyond (falling short of?) masochism, that is, outside the sphere of the subject's sexual quest.

But it is Winnicott, Ferenczi's unavowed disciple, who best explains the latter's innovation in his 1929 text:

> I suggest that the mother hates the baby before the baby hates the mother, and before the baby can know his mother hates him … A mother has to be able to tolerate hating her baby without doing anything about it. She cannot express it to him. If, for fear of what she may do, she cannot hate appropriately when hurt by her child she must fall back on masochism.[8]

It is not only, as Freud said, that hate precedes and conditions love in the act of discovery of the object; to arrive at that hate, the infant must first be the object of the mother-environment, on which he is totally dependent. And at the very beginning, since he is not yet able to hate in response to hate, nor to know that he is hated, the mother-environment must be able to experience her hate without (too much) guilt and without retaliation, without masochistic or sadistic *discharge*. This hate is to be experienced as a natural response to what Winnicott calls "ruthless love"—a stage preliminary to integration.

But how are we to reflect on that which conditions integration in the Winnicottian sense, without reference to the protective function performed by the environment, as Ferenczi saw it in 1929, and as he presented it again in the *Clinical Diary*, in a discussion on the "unprotected child"?

> The unprotected child is ready to be blown up, so to speak. (Link with my little work on children's desire to die). Narcosis, hypnosis, anxiety destroy the synthesizing functions. The feeling of not being loved or of being hated (link with father and mother hypnosis) makes the desire to live, that is, to be unified, disappear. Inability to be alone.[9]

The "inability to be alone"—another concept Winnicott owes to Ferenczi—is rooted in a lack of protection, that is, in an inadequate processing of hate by the parent, a parent unable to be alone with his hate. Protection relies on parental "tact" in adapting to the immaturity of the baby who cannot yet respond to hate with hate. Of course, the inability to be alone can refer to the structural inability to bear alone the Freudian *Hilflösigkeit*, the state of absolute dependence (physical and psychical) of the newborn—inability to be alone, that is, without the parent's narcissistic and libidinal investments.[10] But here, the term refers to the catastrophic obligation to remain alone and closed off in that solitude, without subsequently gaining access to the living and relation-sustaining solitude linked to a confirmed desire to live, and to the willingness to experience a state of desire.

But a preliminary condition must be fulfilled in order for the narcissistic and erotic investments of the parents to grant the infant the narcissistic foundations underlying the desire to live, enabling him to shed existential guilt associated with hate—always dramatically, since, there being no place to direct it, it is inevitably turned against oneself. Here, we are not in the sphere of what Harold Searles calls the baby's desire for revenge, directed towards the mother who takes away the breast.[11] We are, rather, at the heart of the making of a schizophrenic, in this sphere so closely explored by him, in which "the effort to drive the other person crazy" is the equivalent of murder, where the mother threatens to go mad if the child separates from her, where recourse to the child as therapist goes hand-in-hand with the recusal of his help ...[12] No doubt, there is reason to think that this very specific sphere of hate is particularly active in the treatment of borderline patients, at least in the most pronounced forms.[13]

To be saved from such a hellish situation, the newborn must experience the feeling that his physical and psychic functioning are sources of erotic and narcissistic satisfaction for those on whom the satisfaction of his own basic needs depends—when he cannot yet place himself in that position, cannot find a centre in an "inside" under construction. This is how he will be able to "forgive" his arrival, by feeling welcome. This will allow him to discover autoeroticism: the investigation of his own body, in which the pleasure derived from drive satisfaction is equivalent—according to Freud—to the reduction of localisable internal tensions.

Self-investigation must succeed in establishing the pleasure in functioning—the pleasure of being—literally placing self-representation at the heart of the thought process. To arrive at this, the parent first has to bear his own hatred, not only reactive hate prompted by the infant or his "ruthless love," but the hate generated by the child's conception, which inevitably separates him from his parents and reawakens *in him* their hatred of him and his hatred of them—a subjectless hate, as it were, which temporarily confuses the self with the other ... All this is what is missing in the borderline sphere.

* * *

This patient was sent to me by an analyst who had been my analysand; the patient had completed a lengthy analysis with her.[14] Our second preliminary meeting was especially noteworthy, foretelling what was to come; it contrasted with the first meeting in which firmly established hysteria seemed to hold centre stage. After a few minutes, the patient literally dropped to the ground, letting herself slide—spill?—out of the chair to the ground, shaken by more or less restrained sobs and spasms, without speaking. She only pulled herself up when I indicated the end of the session, and she recovered quite easily.

After an initial feeling of shock, I interpreted a sort of battle in myself between two types of interpretive scenes: a highly sexualised scene in which the seductive abandon manifests as a subsidence that gripped my attention; a scene with nobody in it, in which what lay on the floor was a puppet whose strings had been dropped. Long afterwards, I came to see the tension between these two scenes as reflecting the conflict between the development and the erasure of overly invasive countertransferential affects.

Two years later, the second scene became all-pervasive, although I did not feel myself to be the subject of the interpretation—as if there was no one there, either to interpret or to be interpreted. Action took the place of interpretation (of the interpretable); the foretold narcissistic catastrophe took place: several serious suicide attempts occurred, marking the emergence of a melancholic foundation—beyond reactive depression, primarily linked to devastating developments in a (self-)destructive relationship with a man whose depression she was taking charge of, although this depression was firmly denied by the man in question and even by my patient.

Throughout these two years, a story unfolded almost silently, as if in the background or outside the transference, describing a childhood and an adolescence marked by the threat of incest and by cruelly pervasive incestuous mistreatment. The transference took the form of a paradoxical invocation intended to burden me with guilt/free me from guilt: *offering me thanks for being there to listen to her, and reproaching me for not hearing her*. Everything is set down in writing but I can do nothing for her except forgive her for this irreparable mutilation of her being which condemns me and renders psychoanalysis powerless—a condemnation from which she wants to protect me by suggesting, at the start of each session, that we stop the analysis, claiming that it is wasted on her since she is unable to "help herself."

All libidinal investment must be destroyed. The feminine presentation, which at first took the form of a seductive presence, gradually disappeared; henceforth there were only suicidal acts and their consequences, the refuge found in the pseudo rest area[15] offered by hospitalisation and psychotropic drugs, providing the only *relief* possible in the now certain absence of the helpful other. The predominant element in her present analysis was the dramatic undercurrent of a murder to be displayed by being perpetuated *against oneself*, in the absence of someone to kill who could survive the attempt.

At the start of the third year, a dream seemed to indicate a turning point, holding the possible promise of at least partial extrication from the narcissistic trap which forced the patient to do almost nothing except try to discover what prevented the analyst from being a "helpful other."[16]

> *She walks towards a lake with someone. On the surface of the water, she sees a child (one or two years old, more likely a boy) floating with his face in the water. Then the child turns over and looks at her; his gaze is clear and lively. He is no longer in any danger of drowning. She leaves, with the person who came with her, thinking that the child must learn to fend for himself.*

I find it reassuring to think that this scenario indicates an introjective turn in the transference, presuming that there is, on the part of the patient, a recognition—even an investment—of my investment. As if the patient was becoming able to help herself by accepting my help and my interest in her; as if she was, perhaps, starting to feel at least a little of the transformational power of this introjection.

Indeed, the atmosphere of the sessions changed. The transference seemed to reintroduce a minimal libidinal element, with both a libidinal and a narcissistic aspect, which could begin to oppose the rejection of all libidinal investments—the foreseeable end result of self-confinement in narcissistic hate. The body and the face, whose collapse had testified to a strong loss of interest/disassignment, drew themselves up: they recovered by regaining the narcissistic and sexual investments which had been reserved almost exclusively for the words spoken in the sessions, softly—words serving only to testify, powerfully but on the edge of silence, to an unneeded life, an unwelcome existence.

The body and the face drew themselves up: discourse regained its lost advantage over narration, words took on a firmer shape and were spoken in a voice that let itself be heard, instead of fading. The clothing, posture and facial expression above all started to allow the feminine to resume its place.

As the sessions continued, in the months that followed this dream, the evolution of the clinical picture allowed me to take pleasure in thinking again, and to convince myself—even going so far as to authorise the publication of a text describing this experience—that this patient had been the living source of the concentration of theoretical and clinical questions about the status, in the analytic community, of the founding dialogue between Freud and Ferenczi, which was both innovative and brutal. The convincing story of my patient seemed to paint a beautiful picture … Shortly afterwards, she ended this analysis suddenly, having given me no warning signs. I was left in complete uncertainty as to her ability to resist suicidal tendencies.

Now, having finished a second account of this analysis, that is, in the aftermath of the aftermath, I would say that my patient's act of ending the analysis was the staging of a disguising/revealing of her melancholic position, presented as a claim. It was as if she vitally needed to feel *untreatable*, irrevocably condemned to death in the eyes of the other … something I had failed to see. It was as if she had come from the universe of a child *of incest*, that is, a victim of psychic murder without a witness, to bring together in me, in confusion, what was left unanalysed by her first analyst—my ex-analysand—to denounce, by enacting it, the incestuous confusion between what remained unanalysed in the analyst of the previous analyst, and what remained unanalysed in her own analyst: myself in both cases.

What is there to do in the face of this radical form of self-destruction which was first rendered entirely thinkable by Ferenczi in "The Unwelcome Child and His Death-Instinct?" The infant is subjected to the injunction to take on the psychic murder initially carried out by the other on himself—the essential other at the stage of total dependence. This self-destructive submission to a murderous injunction, which produces borderline states with melancholic traits, could be seen as an element of incestual confusion, destined to be *continually* transferred and brought into the present.

This injunction confused the infant's psychic development by introducing an instigation to repeat the devitalisation of any relationship, a compulsion to reduce all relationships to an a-relational connection. The only means to survive an unwitnessed murder is incorporation: the importing of murderous hate, to kill in oneself the need for the other in order to feel alive, as if one was killing one's own self in the other. If the splitting serves adequately as a defensive measure, this murderous hate can, in fact, be used as a means to survive which makes it possible to rescue a degree of libidinal investment just high enough, in the choice of a relation with an other, inevitably condemned to re-enact the dereliction of the helpful other. In any event, this is the path that can lead to a transferential relation to an analyst, if such a relation comes into being.

Be that as it may, to bear this kind of self-hate, to make it possible for patients to bear it, to accompany them in the process needed to redirect it in the transference, the analyst must be able to face his own hate, as Winnicott theorised in "Hate in the Countertransference." What is required of the analyst is to accept what affects him in the inaugural scene of unwelcome arrival, of murderous self-hate that expresses murderous hate of the other, of murderous hate of the other that *contains* murderous self-hate. Without the willingness to accept all this, the transferential redirection of hatred cannot occur, and therefore there can be no symbolisation of the murder.

Accepting oneself in this way is only possible by staying in touch with the expected advent of the pleasure of thinking. What is accepted is the unknown in the transference *and* the subsequent possibility of thinking through a part of it, never definitively established: the possibility of transforming it into a source of thought, enigmatic and unstable, but alive. In this case, for me, the unknown and its aftermath involved the melancholic dimension, with two aspects that must be clearly distinguished. On the one hand, the melancholic aspect of borderline disorders—where absence threatens to summon disappearance—and on the other hand, the melancholic aspect of the enactment of absence by the analyst.

When dealing with borderline functioning, the analyst's enactment of absence risks being *melancholised*. The aim of the treatment will be the attainment of "detachability"[17] by the patient: through the acceptance by the analyst of the obligation to invest his own thought process as a space where the void in the analysand's thinking can be lodged. The borderline sphere activates the analyst's fear of loss, when he tries to render his patient's psychic functioning thinkable. His thoughts appear to be deprived of their ability to symbolise absence, because they are the place where the analysand has deposited his paradoxical need for *self-effacement in the other*. This need is likely to set up a dangerous contest between acting or opposing the injunction to make oneself disappear, a contest whose outcome is supposed to depend completely and exclusively on the analyst.

This very particular type of transferential attribution became clear to me in my work with this patient when I examined frankly, in the aftermath, the internal need that led me to address an audience based on this case, setting aside the shield I usually grant myself by recourse to the literary device of self-writing … This time, I needed not only the support of publication, but more specifically the aftermath of writing and its reiteration, in a form rooted in Freudian writing rather than literature.

* * *

What I wrote was, we might say, a presentation of my "transference on psychoanalysis." But, to conclude, I would like to return to the origins of my reasoning. Ferenczi's analysis with Freud is impossible because it sets up a conflict between: i) an analyst who has not been analysed and cannot bear an analysand with the transferential need to find the absence of this experience an intolerable fault, and ii) an analysand with this transferential need, whose only recourse is to become the analyst of his analyst by reinventing psychoanalysis with and despite him. But this impossible analysis introduces the possibility of a dialogue between psychoanalysts *elsewhere*—but a dialogue naturally threatened from within, as it were, by the displacement of passions.

The dialogue between Freud and Ferenczi, creative and destructive, could generate a transferential scene for every analyst, a scene both original and originary—original: from the beginnings of psychoanalysis; originary: reactivated in and by the functioning of the analyst in his practice, with this reactivation shaping his identity as an analyst. This scene, whose content is, hopefully, unprecedented and particular with each patient, comes alive for the analyst in his internal dialogue, his internal exchange, the playback of his listening. It's not exactly that he speaks to himself in the session; the words that come to him silently keep forming an ever-changing cluster of polarities, keeping him in touch with his resistances and with the source of what he brings to the transference: an offer of transference.

An internal audience is constituted, an internal witness, living and composite, making it at least partially possible to experience the present/absent third party, in the presence/absence of identifications to one's analysts, whose creative intervention may be requested. When dealing with borderline functioning, this is undoubtedly the necessary condition for transforming the murder of shared creativity between two people into the symbolic and symbol-generating murder of the analyst's analyst, *in his absence*. Introducing absence liberates murderous phantasies: a phantasmatic aim for both analysand and analyst, but which must take divergent paths, that the analyst must make clearly distinct and differentiate, in the face of the patient's incestual behaviour.

Freud is an unanalysable analyst whose place as an analyst is occupied and rendered immutable by the invention of psychoanalysis. At the same time, Ferenczi is an unanalysable analysand. While Freud, the inventor of psychoanalysis, excluded the possibility of having an analyst, Ferenczi could only try desperately to reinvent psychoanalysis, so as to make it possible for Freud to be his analyst—Freud, who could not and did not desire to have an analyst. In other words, Ferenczi could only try—and fail—to fill the empty place of his analyst's analyst through theoretical creation, expecting it to accomplish the impossible: to analyse Freud so that Freud could analyse him. The ensuing failure was catastrophic: no one was there to receive the murderous hate of the *unwelcome child-therapist*. This hate was to remain an *undiscussed subject* between them. Ferenczi had no choice but to transform his impossible attribution into a source of creative thought—at a great cost, as we know.

Freud's internal dialogue and his dialogue with Ferenczi, which reflects it, designate a virtual position—that of Freud's analyst. This position, which for Ferenczi stands for an empty place, must be invested by analysts as vacant, not empty. This vacancy is entrusted to them. They must resist the irreducible temptation of filling the position themselves, or have it filled by an idealised figure: a temptation associated with their status as descendants of Freud and heirs to the dialogue between

Freud and Ferenczi. Their task is to continue Freud's internal dialogue, which was taken up by Ferenczi, but to do it differently. To achieve this, they must allow the Freud–Ferenczi dialogue, intrinsically threatened with impossibility, to continue and to remain creative in them, which implies that they consent to conceive of the latent destructivity associated with holding the place of the analyst's analyst, pre-inscribed by the inevitable lack of an analyst for Freud.

The hypothesis of an agency instituting the analyst's transference makes it possible to consider the stakes involved in an offer made by the analyst *as a condition* of the analysand's request. At the same time, each analysis calls forth an original scene: the analyst's relation to the origins of psychoanalysis, to the Freudian beginning and the Ferenczian starting-over. Each of them must consent to a symbolic murder guaranteeing the symbolic power of the Freudian corpus within (and around) the analytic community. In other words, forfeiting the desire to *occupy* the place of the analyst's analyst, left vacant, would guarantee the work of the third party in the *psychoanalytic* thinking of psychoanalysts, as they establish the new beginnings of psychoanalysis with and beyond Freud: the sacrifice of the imaginary third.

The analytic community is both an ideal and a necessary figuration of thirdness, beyond considerations of belonging and the pitfalls of imitation associated with transferential identifications and counter-identifications. It is an additional, demanding element in each analysis, so that the analyst ascertains each time, *in person*, its impossible reenactment.

Notes

1 Ferenczi, S., "The Unwelcome Child and His Death-Instinct," *International Journal of Psycho-Analysis*, 10, 1929: 125–129.
2 Ferenczi, S., "The Unwelcome Child and His Death-Instinct," *International Journal of Psycho-Analysis*, 10, 1929: 125–129.
3 Ferenczi, S., *The Clinical Diary of Sándor Ferenczi*, Dupont, J. (Ed.), Harvard University Press, 1995.
4 Ferenczi, S., "The Unwelcome Child and His Death-Instinct," *International Journal of Psycho-Analysis*, 10, 1929: 125–129.
5 In formulating a qualitative deficit of psychic presence from the perspective of the *infans*, I prefer to use the term "destructive fault" rather than the usual term "failure of the environment," which creates some difficult to solve problems, among them the definition of environment in Winnicott's minimalist perspective: the adaptation needed by the newborn to survive.
6 This reformulation was prompted by the concepts of life narcissism and death narcissism: Green, A., *Life Narcissism Death Narcissism*, Free Association Books, 2001. See, in this regard, Green, A., *On the Destruction and Death Drives*, Levine, H. (Ed.), Karnac, 2023.
7 Green, A., "Death in Life: A Reassessment of the Death Drive," in Guillaumin, J. et al., *L'Invension de la pulsion de mort*, Dunod, 2000, p. 169.
8 Winnicott, D.W., "Hate in the Counter-Transference," *International Journal of Psycho-Analysis*, 30, 1949: 69–74.
9 Ferenczi, S., *The Clinical Diary of Sándor Ferenczi*, Dupont, J. (Ed.), Harvard University Press, 1995, p. 70.

10 To be sure, the Ferenczian notion of a parent could be reconsidered from the more Freudian perspective of plural identifications to the maternal and paternal figures.

11 Searles, H., "The Psychodynamics of Vengefulness," *Psychiatry*, 19, 1956.

12 Searles, H., *Collected Papers on Schizophrenia and Related Subjects*, Routledge, 1986.

13 "It seems to me doubtful whether a human child as he develops is capable of tolerating the full extent of his own hatred in a sentimental environment. He needs hate to hate. If this is true, a psychotic patient in analysis cannot be expected to tolerate his hate of the analyst unless the analyst can hate him ... I believe an analysis is incomplete if even towards the end it has not been possible for the analyst to tell the patient what he, the analyst, *did unbeknown* for the patient whilst he was ill, in the early stages. Until this interpretation is made the patient is kept to some extent in the *position of infant—one who cannot understand what he owes to his mother*" (Winnicott, D.W., "Hate in the Counter-Transference", *International Journal of Psycho-Analysis*, 30, 1949: 69–74).

14 This clinical situation is used here as a case presentation. The situation, which was referred to earlier, literally acted as a pre-text of writing undertaken twice, a process of elaboration with two stages of writing: "Au commencement était le meurtre" (In the Beginning Was the Murder), in *Le Coq Héron*, 224, 2016: 10–20; then in this work, *supra*, and in the present passage.

15 In Winnicott's perspective: an internal space free of any relational demands. The patient speaks of the "asylum" as if it's a "home" which protects her from involvement with others. But this home now has the serious disadvantage of being precarious and temporary, while it had been made *certain*—guaranteed and safe—by the unconditional availability of her previous analyst.

16 I am now using the term as Ferenczi understood it (Ferenczi, S., *The Clinical Diary of Sándor Ferenczi*, Dupont, J. (Ed.), Harvard University Press, 1995). The "fellow human being" is a concept shared by Freud and Ferenczi.

17 We must make a clear distinction between melancholia and the work of melancholia, defined by a quest for "detachability," as Rosenberg defined it: Rosenberg, B., *Masochisme mortifère et massochisme gardien de vie* (Deadly Masochism and Life-Preserving Masochism), PUF, 1991.

Part 3

Writing at the Borderline

Delimiting a space: if a writing project can be specified and described as self-writing, it would be good to inscribe it within the presentation of a space: the space of internal life, presented in writing as an internal scene showing how the author sees himself through what he hears in his words. And when he testifies to his life, a life saved from attempted extermination, his self-presentation reveals a vital effort to hear "beyond survival" in the words.

Aharon Appelfeldt's *The Story of a Life*[1] is perhaps the most explicit description of this effort. The author declares the book to be autobiographical, and constructs it in an unusual manner, centering it on geographical locations. They structure the narration and the arrangement of recollections; self-presentation is literally built on their presentation as they relate to the events and affects associated with them, and not the other way around. Throughout the narration, the description of the places of survival takes up most of the account of what is remembered. The past is only accessible through the body and that which in the body supports words and the voice. Physical places make remembering possible because they testify to survival and thereby allow survivors to find or recover their voice, that is, the "right words" rooted in the body: the words of life beyond survival. In this respect, the book as a whole raises a vital objection, to oppose the "proponents of fact".[2]

Continuing to live must be distinguished from survival and defined as the construction of an expectation, revealed in written material which we shall consider a space where writing is expected. This writing testifies—like a "witness mound," to what remains, what has resisted the recourse to writing which testifies to the overcoming of the harm done to confidence in what is heard in the words spoken to oneself when addressing the other. This confidence presupposes an internal experience of oneself that makes it possible to feel alive and at ease in the world, and sufficiently certain of one's place as a distinct human being among other distinct human beings. This confidence was irrevocably altered by the Holocaust.

We must acknowledge fundamental differences in the testimonial aspect of writing between Imre Kertész and Primo Levi, the two authors who essentially guided and will continue to guide my questioning concerning living beyond survival. Only the latter—in some of his works, particularly *If This Is a Man*—can be said to have deliberately chosen a testimonial modality portraying the surviving witness.

DOI: 10.4324/9781003542483-8

Kertész testifies to his living beyond survival by means of writing, while Levi cannot refrain from testifying as a survivor in his writing. The former's writing confides in the words, to create an interlocutor through the fictionalisation of his erasure, while the latter's writing expects the words to address themselves to an *external* interlocutor.

Still, beyond their differences, their works *testify* to surviving an attack on the need for the other in order to feel oneself exist in *one's own* psychic space. This brings Martin Miller to mind. What these three authors have in common is that each of them in his own way illustrates powerfully the need for intrapsychic reality when it differs from cultural reality, and the need to integrate the latter in order to make it intelligible, through configurations indicating the outdated nature of that reality, as well as its present configurations or changes.

Notes

1 Appelfeld, A., *The Story of a Life: A Memoir*, Schocken, 2004.
2 Chiantaretto, J.-F., "Les limites de l'écriture de soi: à propos de Kertész et Appelfeld," in Chiantaretto, J.-F. (Ed.), *Écritures de soi, écritures des limites*, Hermann, 2014.

Chapter 6

Survival in Words

For a psychoanalyst, reflecting on (and with) psychoanalysis implies considering the culture, and not only the place of psychoanalysis in the culture or the place of culture in psychoanalysis. As Laurence Kahn illustrates in her imaginative book,[1] it is more important than ever to be aware of the effect on psychoanalysis of the hate generated in and by the culture—a question Freud considered in *Civilization and Its Discontents*, and in "Why War." She follows in Freud's footsteps but integrates the fracture introduced by the Holocaust, considered an autoimmune disease of the culture, in the Freudian sense of the word. This fracture brings into question the relationship between language and hate—in its narcissistic and objectal life-and-death forms: from self-hate to hate of the other, from the language of hate to hatred of language as the space of culture.

For over a decade, Imre Kertész has accompanied my "continuing education" in psychoanalysis. He exemplifies most faithfully what I look for in an author's writing: the effect of knowledge promised by the text, that is, to render thinkable for me, through the exchanges between the reader and the author, that which affects me in my patients and which I try to repress more or less temporarily, using the very words of psychoanalysis—knowing, of course, that a writer belongs to no one, not even to himself: he cannot be reduced to any presentation, his own or that of his reader, even if he is a psychoanalyst!

Kaddish for an Unborn Child, in particular, enabled me to read Kertész's writing as a vitally needed place of exile, to resist the self-destructiveness inherent in survival. In my view, this author's writing transforms self-destructiveness into energy and, at the same time, into literary material in the construction of the aftermath of the experience of the Nazi camps. "The culture of Auschwitz," as he calls it, raises a crucial question: is it not the case that culture after the Holocaust should be considered *as well* from the perspective of its participation in the self-destructivity of the human species? Thanks to the unique resources he can bring to examining this question, I found that Kertész's writing provided a better approach to what I call internal interlocution, that is, the inner experience of the self in words acting as potential witnesses of the identificatory constellation: potential witnesses of the others in oneself, confronting the subject with internal alterity, that of the other as well as one's own. The aim is to establish the conditions necessary to articulate a

DOI: 10.4324/9781003542483-9

psychoanalytic approach to writing and to the psychopathology of borderline situations, seen as a transnosographic mode of rethinking—not as a new nosographic entity.[2]

* * *

Thinking about Auschwitz is inextricably connected with Imre Kertész;[3] to be more exact, to the presence of Auschwitz in each of us after the Holocaust, precisely in the place where the intrapsychic reality of the individual subject is only accessible through its intrication with cultural reality. And keeping in mind that all of Kertész's work is an assertion that Auschwitz must be subjected to thought, and is perhaps only thinkable starting from its destructive presence in individual psychic functioning—which gives Auschwitz its universal dimension.

While in *The Rebel* Camus states Bolshevism tends towards universality, contrary to Nazism or fascism, Kertész points out Nazism's demand for universality through destruction, negation, "hatred and murder."[4] When Kertész uses the expression "Nazi counterculture," he is certainly referring to Nazi hatred of culture, which is attacked for being the space of communal life, that is, the space of the human in *each individual*. But above all, what is upheld is a perspective inherited from Freud and taken up again by Adorno: Nazism goes to extremes in its hatred of culture, a hatred produced and reinforced by the culture itself.[5] Indeed, we might ask if Kertész goes further than the author of *Civilization* ... when he advances the idea of a "culture of Auschwitz." Kertész, like Adorno, sees the negation of culture as a component of the negativity intrinsically at work in culture, but in addition to this, he asserts that awareness of this negativity is a new value made possible by Auschwitz.[6]

The "culture of Auschwitz": to destroy the Jews means destroying European values. "Auschwitz and everything pertaining to it (and what does not pertain to it henceforth?) is the greatest trauma that has befallen European man since the Crucifixion."[7] The extermination of the Jews enacted the self-hatred of the Western world. This idea is helpful for grasping what Kertész calls atonal language, the only language that can express what Auschwitz did to culture: it annihilated hate as we understood it in pre-Auschwitz language. Kertész refers to Jean Améry when he writes:

> I am quoting the words of authors who have bequeathed to us the true experiences of the Holocaust and are already speaking a post-Auschwitz language. What sort of language is that? Borrowing a technical term from music for my own purposes, I have dubbed it atonal language ... In literature too a tonic keynote once existed, a set of values based upon a generally accepted morality of ethics, that defined the system of relationships among statements and ideas. The few who risked their existence to bear witness to the Holocaust knew that the continuity of their lives had been torn asunder, that it wasn't possible for them to go on with their lives ... in the manner that society requires, and to formulate their experiences in the pre-Auschwitz language.[8]

He also speaks of Thomas Mann, a different kind of author altogether:

> To write an atonal novel. What is the novel's tonality? A distinct *basso continuo*, a fundamental note resonating throughout the text. Does such a fundamental note exist? If it does, it has run dry. Thus, it is to write a novel without a definite moral, with only the original forms of the experience—experience in the literal and mysterious sense of the word.[9]

This would inscribe Kertész in the lineage of Freud and Adorno, based on the idea of a pact between barbarism and culture.[10] But Kertész considers the Freudian idea of originary parricide as belonging to pre-Auschwitz culture, and therefore stripped of legitimacy:

> It is not Freud who taught us that we must fear ourselves because we don't know what we might or might not be capable of doing, but our own experience … To learn that the guilt produced by the originary parricide created a culture would bring tears to our eyes if so many fathers, sons, daughters and mothers had not been murdered since then, if we did not see that no one feels remorse, and that all this has not made us more intelligent.[11]

This is the perspective from which Kertész considers the question of fate, a question central to his work. He sees it as the locus of an ambiguity in his manner of identifying himself as a Jewish writer:

> If I say: "I am a Jewish writer (because that fact most of all stamped and stamps its mark on my circumstances), then I have not said that I myself am Jewish—because sadly, by virtue of my culture and convictions, I cannot say that. But I can say that I am a writer of the *Galut*, the exile, an anachronistic Jewish mode of existence, a chronicler of its liquidation, messenger of its necessary discontinuation. The *Endlösung* plays a decisive role in this respect; anyone for whom that experiment at exterminating the Jews, Auschwitz, is his sole Jewish identity, in a certain sense cannot after all be called a Jew."[12]

What Kertész means by "fatelessness" (the title of his semi-autobiography) is a loss of the individual's personal responsibility. But this loss cannot be experienced as an individual loss, because it concerns a collective condition. As indicated by the German term *unschuldig*, this loss designates innocence: one is not responsible for oneself and is thus faultless and free of guilt. But how are we to conceive the destiny allotted by the Nazis to the Jews: to be superfluous, literally destined to be "liquidated," in Kertész terminology? So-called assimilated Jews were particularly threatened with seeing their Jewishness reduced to nothing more than the object of the Nazi extermination project. This caused Kertész to consider a question inspired by Kierkegaard: in this context, should we speak of a "community of fate" or of a "community of fatelessness"?[13]

The survivors are left with a paradoxical task: to emerge from accidental survival, from the condemnation to innocence, in order to attain personal failure and responsibility.[14] Indeed, we would do well to re-examine in this light the generally so poorly posed question of the supposed guilt of the survivor. How is Oedipus to address himself at the height of tragedy? How do the determinants of fate intersect with tragic conflict?

But while the survivor of Nazi camps cannot escape the vital obligation of searching for a personal solution to fatelessness, although this solution is more or less impossible to find, the "functional man" is doomed to settle into fatelessness. *Galley-Boat Log* makes this explicitly clear: the "functional man," the "new man," an ideological product of Nazism and to some extent Stalinism, is a man of the masses, without qualities, deprived of a connection between existing and being, predetermined and reducible to an assigned role.[15]

> The reality of a functional man is a pseudo-reality, a life-replacing life … Indeed, his life is mostly a tragic process or error, but without the necessary tragic consequences … No one lives his own reality that way, only his function without the existential experience of his life, without his own fate. This could mean the subject of work for him.[16]

Kertész insists on differentiating between being a Jewish writer and being a Jew in order to lay claim to writing as his place, the place of exile where he has chosen to exist, to come into his own being, to create or build his fate. In other words, for him, writing is the tragic place where he can experience himself as an enigma,[17] where he can make use of tragic conflict: "My ambition as a writer: to write something that kills me."[18] Writing is a vital function;[19] it creates a place of self-observation making it possible to experience being two in one and thereby avoiding the "impersonal fate" of the "functional man": "At last, I was able to escape this impersonal fate; my greatest adventure, after all, is myself. I conceived of myself and built myself. Against all odds."[20]

Writing is a place freely chosen, never naturally given, making it possible to render representable the absence of free choice, imposed *as if naturally* by totalitarian ideologies. This ideology is presented as such under communism, and closely represents the new man promised by the Nazi project. Its updated version threatens contemporary "mass democracy,"[21] even in today's liberal democracies where ideological rigidification is gaining ground through the dominance of communication and the elimination of *dis-sensus*. The assessment of functional man can be extended to Western society as a whole, which tends to set in place a transparent, horizontal world, with functionality as an immanent trait and ideology as the means of consensual totalisation, played down in all discourse or narrative. The totalitarian reduction of the reality of the world to a purely ideological concept presumes that objective reality exists independently of us. This Marxist dogma explains not only totalitarian ideology, but adherence to the principle of ideology itself, which reduces the world to an idea. It is from this point of view that we can understand the importance of the figure of Cain, the sign of the need for transcendence expressed in Kertész's diaries:

> Man is immersed in constant discourse, signs and dialogue; all his gestures and expressions. And because he is constantly "expressing himself," he needs to address someone, who ultimately could be God. The great flow of Human Narration in which we are all seeking our place. We all live under a Gaze. A Gaze that takes us into account. A person not taken into account is in distress.

> … The darkness of total distress begins with the absence of a Gaze, the feeling of being disregarded. This is what Cain felt.[22]

* * *

Contrary to Primo Levi, who became a writer as an outcome of Auschwitz, Kertész attributes the start of his activity as a writer to the strangeness of his life in communist Hungary, which protected him from disillusionment and the temptation of suicide to which survivors in democratic societies succumbed.

> I was helped [kept from suicide] over the course of the past decades by a "society" that, following Auschwitz, amply demonstrated through the form of so-called Stalinism that there could be no question of freedom, liberation, catharsis, etc.—none of the things that intellectuals and philosophers in more fortunate climates not only spoke of but also clearly believed in.

> I was trapped in a society that guaranteed me the continued life of a prisoner, thereby also excluding the possibility of erring. This is clearly why I was not engulfed by the high tide of disappointments that overwhelmed those who had similar experiences but who found themselves living in more open societies, the rising waters first splashing at their feet as they tried to flee, then slowly rising to their throats.[23]

This strangeness of the stranger saved him from the *impersonalisation* characterising the "functional man," although his psychic malleability predisposed him to it. A few years after Kertész returned from Buchenwald, when he became a prison guard, he was able to imagine the position of the executioner and he started to write a novel left unfinished, *I, the Executioner*. A fragment of it, attributed to one of his ghostwriters, was reproduced in *Fiasco*.[24]

I would add that the feeling of strangeness, evident in the author's diaries as well as in his fiction, persisted throughout his life, from his chaotic childhood all through the communist and post-communist eras in Hungary, *and* his experience in Auschwitz and Buchenwald—a strangeness presented without pathos, accompanied by the explicit disavowal of any testimonial posture in regard to traumatic experience. In Kertész's writing, traumatic experience is not present as such, as an external, objectifiable reality separate from the writing: it is literally inseparable from its portrayal in writing.

It is a matter of "surviving one's survival," as well as avoiding the emotional danger associated with testimony. The ending of *The Last Inn* takes the form of an open letter which asserts:

> I think I have produced a literary oeuvre that can be considered a testimony of conscience and solidarity with the victims and survivors among whom I count myself. At the same time, my work can be considered a personal accomplishment. By writing about Buchenwald, I transcended Buchenwald, I freed myself of my own Buchenwald. Ever since I experienced Buchenwald the first time, and then brought it to life as an imaginary world, as literature, for me Buchenwald has become a kind of abstraction that I must approach with caution. To present myself as a real witness to real events, as a "war veteran" in Semprun's words, as a former victim, would mean reliving things I have left behind, returning to the real Buchenwald; in short, it would force me to make an emotional effort so intense that asking me to do this is not possible.[25]

Indeed, writing saves the writer from the *presence* of the camp by making it possible for him to imagine it, in the social and cultural context of the writing, that of communist Hungary. The camp must be reduced to a literary text, as if it was only possible to survive an imaginary camp—by oneself for others and, perhaps and differently, through others. One year later, Kertész went back to this idea, already discussed in *Galley-Boat Log*, to emphasise its importance, indissociably ethical and vital:

> The obligation to survive accustoms us to falsify, if at all possible, the criminal reality in which we find ourselves, while the duty to remember urges us to introduce in our memories a sort of consolation, the balm of self-pity and self-glorification of the victims.[26]

The battle between the obligation to survive and the duty to remember finds concrete expression in the fight between the work of writing and the work of remembering. Kertész is absolutely determined to be the author of his life, which no doubt explains the fact that in the last part of his work, after the onset of Parkinson's disease (2000) and after receiving the Nobel Prize (2002), he noted that he was torn between the writing of diaries and the writing of fiction.[27] Until then, with the exception of *Fatelessness*, his novels had been able to depict the fictional decomposition of the self, through fictionalised doubles—in *Fiasco*—or through the fictional construction of an internal dialogue that turns into a soliloquy—In *Kaddish for an Unborn Child*. Now, the essay or the diary entered into conflict with writing fiction—a conflict resolved by the use of fictionalised doubles in the diary, making the play between the first and the third person more complex, and recourse to self-citation constant.

The aim was to create a viewpoint from which the author-narrator could always watch himself writing, while he observed himself in what he wrote. At the same time, overwhelmed by the shock produced by both the Nobel Prize and the illness, he seemed to overinvest in *Dossier K*: the complete rewriting of auto-biographical interviews initially conducted by his German editor, transformed into a fictionalised interlocutor, to create a work he called a "veritable autobiography"—although this claim does not abolish all ambivalence.[28] In 2014, in *The Last Inn*, Kertész describes *Dossier K*, published in 2006, as the advance remedy for the later work, which he calls a "diary of death,"[29] in which he himself is the fictionalised *I*.

The fact that for Kertész writing is the place and condition of life, is no doubt the main reason for his anger at Adorno's famous proclamation,[30] although he otherwise admires the thinker: "If I may give a straight answer, I consider that statement to be a moral stink bomb that needlessly pollutes the air that is already rank enough."[31]

It might be said that Kertész speaks in bad faith, since he contributes, strangely, to the instrumentalisation of Adorno's phrase by the "professional humanists" whom they both oppose—professional humanists whom Kertész considers murderers because they deny the irreparable refutation of humanism by Auschwitz.

But aside from his anger, Kertész is defending the vital need to write, in the face of the impossibility of writing. He defines himself as a Jewish writer who writes in Hungarian; but he feels compelled to protest against his exile in the Hungarian language, culture and society, as well as against totalitarian *impersonalisation* and Stalinian ideology. This enables him to survive his survival in the Nazi camps, by displacement.

> … as I began writing, I began … to write about Auschwitz in the extended present. The Holocaust and the state of being in which I wrote about the Holocaust bonded indissolubly with one another. Paradoxical as it may sound, my freedom as a writer was not restricted in the communist dictatorship.[32]

This is writing in the aftermath, but carried out in a very particular manner which makes it possible to consider the traumatic experience from another place: relying on the defences and the creativity required to adapt to this aftermath—to adapt by separating from it, by creating the choice of exile. The "Jewish writer who writes in Hungarian" is also a "Western writer writing in Hungarian,"[33] neither truly Jewish, nor truly Hungarian. In fact, it was in Germany[34] that he was recognised as a writer, in the country at the centre of European culture, whose very language testifies to the integration of the Jews—but which is just as indisputably the nation which took radical action to express the self-hatred present in the culture, and whose extermination programmes were aimed at the *disintegration* of the Jews.

Kertész acknowledges the impossibility of writing by fictionalising writing through his identity games, his doubles in self-interviews, and all the modalities of *mise en abyme* of internal dialogue. To do this, he brings three elements together: his own disappearance as an assimilated Jew; the disappearance threatening European culture with the massification of democracies, as an extension of Nazism and Stalinism; and his participation in a European literature of disappearance, predicted by Nietzsche and embodied by Kafka as its most eminent representative.[35] Kertész is familiar with Celan's work, but he radically rejects Semprun's work and even more that of Primo Levi, whom he severely criticises for having retained as his frame of reference the pre-Auschwitz humanist language and culture to testify about Auschwitz.

> If they ask me about Primo Levi again—a mediocre writer, by the way—I'll say that our books—his and mine—take place in different time periods. His book is set *before* Auschwitz and depicts Auschwitz; my book is set after Auschwitz and talks about the *consequences* of Auschwitz.[36]

Kertész does not try to recount or describe Auschwitz, only to make it imaginable. To make imaginable the *inconceivable* deprivation of fate that the camp renders possible: by means of mass assassination and its modalities, which revoke the victims' human status (the industrialisation of killing, the technocratic management of the camps and the transports, the so-called medical experiments, etc.). This fatelessness persists in the survivors after the experience of powerlessness in the camps.

At the end of *Fatelessness*, Kertész declares that "even there," in the Nazi camps, "next to the chimneys, in the intervals between the torments, there was something that resembled happiness."[37] This is only very secondarily a provocation addressed to the professional humanists he accuses of wanting to kill him with their good intentions and their deadly ignorance of evil, irreducible and irreparable. By doing this, Kertész lays claim to the emotional and affective limits of his personal work of remembrance, the inalienable singularity of his experience as the foundation of personal responsibility for his life, gained or regained by writing; but, above all, he lays claim to the transformative power of writing. Still, to take the measure of the vital importance of separating life from writing, and to understand why the experience of the camps is not unrepresentable, but *indescribable*, it is crucial to add that the modification that writing imprints on experience implies that writing is altered by this experience. Writing only captures and isolates traumatic experience if it can transform it by transforming itself, and if it makes life strangely liveable by rendering it relatable.[38] Because it can bear the fragmentation and dispersion of the I, as a failure of the cohesive force of libidinal investments, autoerotic and objectal, and bear to make this failure thinkable and let these investments serve to bring about self-effacement—as is the case in *Kaddish*—writing offers the possibility of sublimating self-liquidation.

Sublimating self-liquidation, *transforming* it into self-multiplication, with narcissistic and libidinal investments in the ego, by means of the various identity games devised by the author-narrator, in what I persist in defining as self-writing. In other words, the written formulation—referring to the author himself—of the self-reflexivity at the core of the inner experiencing of self in the words. That is to say, experiencing the distance between self and oneself, *elsewhere*, in the distance between myself and I; or perhaps, experiencing internal alterity, the two-in-one in what I call internal dialogue, in the context established by the concept of "internal witness."[39]

The "negative hero" of *Fatelessness*, defined by the author as an initiation novel in reverse, is the only kind of hero who can embody cultural negativity and surmount it,[40] by avoiding the trap of self-narration and explanatory narrative. Thus, Kertész's writing takes Goethe's *Truth and Poetry* as an anti-model. Contrary to Goethe, whose autobiography describes a particularly favourable constellation presiding over his birth, Kertész's arrival was poorly timed:

> Well then, at the time I came into the world the Sun was standing in the greatest economic crisis the world had ever known … a party leader by the name of Adolf Hitler looked exceedingly inamicably upon me from amidst the pages of his book *Mein Kampf*, the first of Hungary's Jewish laws, the so-called *Numerus Clausus*, stood at its culmination before its place was taken by the remainder. Every earthly sign … attested to the superfluousness—indeed, the irrationality— of my birth. On top of which, I arrived as a nuisance for my parents: they were on the point of divorcing.[41]

When the arrival of the superfluous being is inscribed in the universal birth register, there is a break in the "spirit of storytelling,"[42] a term Kertész borrowed from Thomas Mann to designate the gaze in which we are held, which survived the Nietzschean announcement of God's death. But after the Holocaust and totalitarianism, it is to atonal language that Kertész assigns the mission of thwarting the inherence proclaimed by ideology. In his view, the ideology can be countered by the refusal to identify with oneself, by rejecting identificatory language and learning to hear the equivocal and the ambiguous at the heart of language—what the words know about things we don't know.[43]

This is why classifying Kertész's identity games as autofiction would be a serious error. His writing is the construction of a "spiritual home"[44] which materialises the beyond: a perspective on life without which life would not be liveable. To make the impossible narration of life relatable makes it possible to experience its enigmatic, elusive truth, its irreducible tragic tension, that must be reconquered after Auschwitz to save it from mere survival. This conquest must take place in the here and now, through the confrontation with the presence of Auschwitz.

I would like to end this discussion with what Georges Didi-Huberman wrote in a book about his confrontation with what remains in Auschwitz of the camp. *Bark* is a commentary on four photographs of the gas chamber taken by a member of the *Sonderkommando*. Three of them are on display at the Auschwitz Museum, without any mention of the position of the photographer, who must have been hiding when he took the photographs. The comment, which protests against the proclaimed *evidence* of the unrepresentable, criticises this exclusion of the photographer in the museum, by referring to the birch trees on the edge of the camp as "silent witnesses" through their bark.

We can think of the surface as that which falls from things: that which comes directly from them, that which is detached from them, what they result in. And that which is detached from them to lay before us, under our gaze, like shreds of a tree bark.[45]

Notes

1 Kahn, L., *What Nazism Did to Psychoanalysis*, Routledge, 2022.
2 See Chiantaretto, J.-F., *Trouver en soi la force d'exister*, Campagne Première, 2011.
3 The reader is referred to the discussion with Laurence Kahn on Kertész at the conference "Psychoanalysis: Analysis of Its Modernity" (based on Laurence Kahn's work), Cerisy-la-Salle, July 2018. See "Survivre/penser: l'écriture de Kertész *pour* le psychoanalyste," in Bombarde, O., Matha, C., and Neau, F. (Eds.), *Quelques motifs de la psychanalyse. À partir des travaux de Laurence Kahn*, Les Belles Lettres, 2020.
4 Kertész, I., *The Holocaust as Culture*, Cooper, T. (Trans.), Seagull Books, 2012.
5 See Kahn, L., *What Nazism Did to Psychoanalysis*, Routledge, 2022.
6 On this point, see Kertész, I., *Sauvegarde* (The Last Inn), Actes Sud, 2012 and "La Culture d'Auschwitz," in *L'Holocauste comme culture*, 2012.
7 Kertész, I., *Journal de galère*, Actes Sud, 2010, p. 32.
8 Kertész, I., *The Holocaust as Culture*, Cooper, T. (Trans.), Seagull Books, 2012.
9 Kertész, I., *Journal de galère*, Actes Sud, 2010, p. 67 (TN: My translation).
10 Kahn, L., *What Nazism Did to Psychoanalysis*, Routledge, 2022.
11 Kertész, I., *Journal de galère*, Actes Sud, 2010, pp. 140–141 (TN: My translation).
12 Kertész, I., "The Diaries of Imre Kertész", excerpts from *The Last Inn* (1 January to 17 November 2001), Literary Hub website, lithub.com.
13 Kertész, I., *The Holocaust as Culture*, Cooper, T. (Trans.), Seagull Books, 2012.
14 See Kahn, L., "Tout naturellement," *Libres cahiers pour la psychanalyse*, 24, 2011, p. 162.
15 Kertész, I., *Journal de galère*, Actes Sud, 2010, p. 11.
16 Kertész, I., *Journal de galère*, Actes Sud, 2010, p. 12.
17 Kertész, I., *Journal de galère*, Actes Sud, 2010, p. 71.
18 Kertész, I., *Journal de galère*, Actes Sud, 2010, p. 68.
19 Kertész, I., *Journal de galère*, Actes Sud, 2010, p. 174.
20 Kertész, I., *Journal de galère*, Actes Sud, 2010, p. 148.
21 Kertész, I., *Sauvegarde* (The Last Inn), Actes Sud, 2012.
22 Kertész, I., *Journal de galère*, Actes Sud, 2010 (TN: My translation).
23 Kertész, I., *The Holocaust as Culture*, Cooper, T. (Trans.), Seagull Books, 2012, pp. 72–73.
24 Clara Royer points out how clearly this unfinished text associates the source of writing with the deep need to understand what leads to mass crimes, rather than what leads to testimony about deportation. Royer, C., *Imre Kertész: "L'histoire de mes morts,"* Actes Sud, 2017, p. 94.
25 Kertész, I., *Sauvegarde* (The Last Inn), Actes Sud, 2012, pp. 222–223.
26 Kertész, I., *The Holocaust as Culture*, Cooper, T. (Trans.), Seagull Books, 2012.
27 This is the conflict described in *The Last Inn* (*L'Ultime Auberge*, Actes Sud, 2015; for instance, p. 185 or p. 218).
28 Kertész, I., *Dossier K: A Memoir*, Wilkinson, T. (Trans.), Melville House, 2013.
29 Kertész, I., *Dossier K: A Memoir*, Wilkinson, T. (Trans.), Melville House, 2013.

30 "To write poetry after Auschwitz is barbaric": Theodor W. Adorno, "Cultural Criticism and Society" (1949). Adorno subsequently went back on this statement several times: in different courses given in 1965, collected in Adorno, T., *Metaphysics: Concept and Problems*, Stanford University Press, 2002; and later in Adorno, T., *Negative Dialectics*, Routledge, 1990. What he means to question is the possibility, after Auschwitz, of poetry as affirmation of life.

31 Kertész, I., *Dossier K: A Memoir*, Wilkinson, T. (Trans.), Melville House, 2013.

32 The essays collected in *The Holocaust as Culture* deal with these questions, in particular "The Freedom of Self-Definition" and "Language in Exile" (Hinchman, L.P., Trans.).

33 Royer, C., *Imre Kertész: "L'histoire de mes morts,"* Actes Sud, 2017, p. 281.

34 Kertész I., *L'Holocauste comme culture*, Actes Sud, 2009, p. 267.

35 This declaration of affiliation is especially meaningful knowing that Kertész is deeply attached to pre-catastrophe European literature, from Goethe to Thomas Mann, with its painfully clairvoyant perspective.

36 Kertész, I., *Sauvegarde*, Actes Sud, 2012, p. 287 (TN: My translation).

37 Kertész, I., *Fatelessness*, Vintage Books, 2004, p. 262.

38 Chiantaretto, J.-F., *Trouver en soi la force d'exister*, Campagne Première, 2011.

39 Chiantaretto, J.-F., *Le Témoin interne*, Aubier, 2005.

40 Kahn, L., *Ce que le nazisme à fait à la psychanalyse*, PUF, 2018, p. 225.

41 Kertész, I., *Fiasco*, Wilkinson, T. (Trans.), Melville House, 1988, p. 91.

42 Kertész, I., *The Holocaust as Culture*, Cooper, T. (Trans.), Seagull Books, 2012.

43 See Laurence Kahn's remarkable discussion on the subject, in Khan, L., *Faire parler le destin*, Klincksieck, 2005, pp. 226–227.

44 Kertész, I., *Galley-Boat Log*, unpublished diaries.

45 Didi-Hubermann, G., *Bark*, Martin, S.E. (Trans.), MIT Press, 2017.

Chapter 7

Writing for...[1]

Primo Levi's *If This Is a Man* testifies in the strongest terms to the inextricable relation between the need to speak to oneself, and the need for another in order to hear oneself. This relation is shown to be a vital necessity for survivors who bear witness, as it is for each of us, to the extent that it can be experienced (we might say "tested"). This, in fact, is the difficulty encountered by readers of this work: to understand the unique specificity of the traumatic injury to this vital need of the survivors who bear witness.

When Primo Levi explains that the experiences described in *If This Is a Man* "wrote themselves"[2] when he returned from Auschwitz, his formulation undoubtedly reflects his premonition that the picture of traumatic solitude would develop in the writing. An incurable solitude: the only cure—whose impossibility he was made to see in the 1980s, with the emergence of revisionism and Holocaust denial—being that humanity as a whole, *as one man*, speak up to legitimate in the aftermath the survivor's internal battle, his determination to speak to himself and to continue imagining the other, in a situation where everything has been put in place to destroy him.

Levi would try, at least after the second edition of *If This Is a Man*, with greater and greater difficulty—perhaps desperately—in the works that followed, to maintain the hope of salvation obtained through writing. In his case, writing is born of survival and contributes to survival: the need to tell the story is presented as life-saving. "I write precisely because I am a chemist": Levi considered that his training allowed him to use writing as a way of taking the inner position of an observer, making it possible to live through the traumatic experience as if it were the catastrophic exploration of an intermediary zone: the inhuman in the human. But how could he bear, as a surviving witness, to testify *in person* to the attack on the human as a constitutive element of the human species?

This is probably the most obvious explanation for the title *If This Is a Man*. And this is where the "immediate, violent impulse to tell the story,"[3] claimed by Levi to have seized hold of him, forces us to view the ethical stakes of testimony from the most difficult angle, the one most likely to inherent passion, the *impossible* question, not of forgiveness, but of the possibility of forgiveness. This question will be re-examined from the partial but essential perspective of the *psychical conditions*

DOI: 10.4324/9781003542483-10

needed for allowing the subject of a traumatic experience to face the possibility of forgiving *or not*—and more specifically, when the trauma could result in the *disappearance* of the other, reanimating the abandonment by the *helpful other*. This type of trauma is a more or less direct attack on the status of "fellow human being." Since the most radical form of this attack, the Holocaust, was a negation of membership in the human species, the *surviving witness* is left with the question of whether he is able to make himself the subject of *his* traumatic experience—to overcome his deposition from the status of human subject, his exclusion, as a fellow human, from among other fellow humans.

Psychical conditions for the possibility of forgiveness: before looking at Levi's view of this question, some general remarks may be useful. Too often challenged or used to achieve more or less ideological aims, this question can be examined from a relational or social perspective by a single individual in regard to another single individual or a group, or by a group in relation to another group or a larger social entity. In all situations, from the strictly individual to the collective, both the individual psyche and the culture are involved, in the sense of Freud's concept of the work of culture (*Kulturarbeit*).

Here we would do well to refer to Nathalie Zaltzman's approach.[4] *Kulturarbeit*, as the "collective guarantor of individual narcissism," provides a "common libidinal space," guarantees in and for each individual a "minimal narcissistic capital," a "minimal certainty of existence for the other."[5] In this sense, *Kulturarbeit* refers to the intrapsychic dimension of the human feeling of belonging, at the very place where the Holocaust has attacked it.

The collapse of that which guaranteed to everyone, unbeknownst to them, unconsciously, the certainty of the existence of a pact between a man and his own self and others—this collapse has taken place, no matter how strong our desire to deny it: for those who were victims of it and did not survive it, for those still alive, and for at least two generations born afterwards. This collapse is now part of all of us.[6]

Testifying to living on implies holding a literally untenable position, condemning the subject of the testimonial act to expose his subjectivity as both the place of this collapse and the place of internal resistance to it. Still, it is in its being given, more than in what it states, that the testimonial act makes readable the intrapsychic dimension of the collective catastrophe, and addresses us as subjects responsible for the human, in each of us and for us all. For "it is through the individual psyche that *Kulturarbeit* is accomplished."[7] And this is where we encounter the question of the possibility of forgiveness, necessary *and* impossible.

To what extent can this question be considered in relation to the Holocaust? As soon as we leave the strictly individual register, the conditions necessary for the presence of a third, and thus the possibility of forgiveness, go radically beyond agreement between two subjects, as is made possible by a sufficiently shared recognition of the fault and its effects, combined with the regret expressed by one and accepted by the other. More radically, in the case of a genocide, does the question of the possibility of forgiveness have any legitimacy?

If forgiveness supposes that someone asks for forgiveness, someone grants it and someone accepts it,[8] in this situation who asks, who grants and who accepts? There exists an inevitable lack of clarity about the identity of the author of the harm, and about the gap between the latter and those who receive the forgiveness: the Nazis, their descendants, Germans of the Nazi period and/or their descendants, the German State? Levi, like all survivors, is haunted by the problem of the gap between those who did not come back from the Nazi camps and those who came back and who cannot speak in the name of the dead and, less still, forgive in their place.

The question of forgiveness seems out of order when the crime is not only collective, but attacks the definition of the human, the presence of the human in each individual. For in a genocide the aim is not only mass murder, but murder carried out in a manner intended to erase the human affiliation of a human group and each of its members. The negation of the human in each victim is clearly a "crime against humanity," beyond human rights and the protection of individuals. To kill a human being considered non-human is potentially an attack on all of us, on each person as a unique representative of the species, representable only to the collectivity of fellow humans, past, present and future: a different fellow human being among fellow humans different from him.

Speaking of Nazi crimes, Levi asserts: "The verb forgive is not in my vocabulary."[9] And he goes on to clarify his position:

> I learned a few years ago that Amery ... defined me as "the forgiver." I consider this neither insult nor praise but imprecision. I am not inclined to forgive, I never forgave our enemies of that time, nor do I feel I can forgive their imitators in Algeria, Vietnam, the Soviet Union, Chile, Argentina, Cambodia and South Africa, because I know of no human act that can erase a crime.[10]

For Levi, to survive means to understand, understand how the crime perpetrated by the Germans could have come about. To understand, but not in order to forgive, but "understand to judge":

> I have been trying for forty years to understand the Germans. To understand how what happened could have happened has been one of my life's goals ... Indiscriminate forgiveness ... is not acceptable to me. "I absolve thee" has no precise meaning for me. I don't believe that anyone, not even a priest, has the power to bind and release ... Whoever commits a crime must pay for it, unless he repents. But this does not mean in words only. A verbal repentance is not enough. I am prepared to release whoever can show through his actions that he is no longer the person he was. And he must not wait too long.[11]

To understand is to risk simplifying, and thus erasing what was done, erasing the responsibility for the murder. But to understand is also to find a bearable solution thanks to which renouncing hate does not mean agreeing to erasure. And to understand by appealing to third parties, such as witnesses are at a trial, is perhaps to seek a manner of confrontation making it possible to survive this terrifying paradox: that the Nazi project of dehumanisation of the victims—the negation of their belonging to the human species—was conceived and carried out by human beings, that is, by fellow beings. But how to accept—at what price?—*to find someone among the Germans who asks for forgiveness?*

When faced with a genocide, evaluating the conditions for the possibility of forgiveness and the limits of the forgivable requires evaluating the possibility and viability of collective procedures involving in one way or another humanity as a whole, in order to recognise that what took place did take place, and concerns every human being *at the present time.* And collective national and international agencies must be authorised to guarantee that someone will ask for forgiveness *and* that there will be someone to judge whether the request can be received—which presupposes that there is someone who can decide what cannot be repaired. This references the legal notion of "Crimes against humanity," regardless of the manner in which it is applied.

But perhaps the main mission of such collective agencies would be to make possible or validate in the aftermath what is most essential: that is, what in the final analysis can only take place on an individual level, in the confrontation between two subjects. The relation involved is that between a repentant subject asking for forgiveness in the present, for himself and for those he represents, and a subject who can grant or not this forgiveness, in his own name and the names of those he represents. Although the Nazis' crime against humanity is unforgivable and cannot be repaired, the possibility of forgiveness insofar as it concerns future generations involves not only the Germans and the Western World, but humanity as a whole, that is, once again, all human beings of the past, the present and the future.

* * *

I repress hatred even within myself. I prefer justice. I have deliberately assumed the calm and sober language of the witness ...; only in this way does a witness in matters of justice perform his task, which is that of preparing the ground for the judge. The judges are my readers. All the same, I would not want my abstaining from explicit judgment to be confused with indiscriminate pardon. No, I have not forgiven any of the culprits, nor am I willing to forgive a single one of them, unless he has shown (with deeds, not words, and not too long afterwards) that he has become conscious of the crimes and errors of Italian and foreign Fascism and is determined to condemn them, uproot them, from his conscience and from that of others ... because an enemy who sees the error of his ways ceases to be an enemy.[12]

Levi's hesitation could perhaps be formulated as follows: *to create the possibility of someone who is asking for forgiveness, even if someone to forgive cannot be found.* This could create the possibility of being the subject of a traumatic experience, in the Holocaust and despite it, in and despite the confrontation with the Nazi project of dehumanisation of the victims, along with mass murder and soul murder.

This interpretation of Levi's writing prompts a reassessment of the *negative* approach to trauma, as proposed by Ferenczi and Winnicott. In that perspective, the lack of psychic inscription of the experience is what paradoxically endows trauma with extreme weight. Trauma always involves psychic mutilation, imposed on the subject by the psychical absence of the other, who disappeared from the very place where the subject needs him—he is gone and unable to recognise the self-effacement at the origin of his disappearance for the subject.

There is no one to recognise the disappearance, and the subject of this failing disappears, ruthlessly innocent, leaving the *subject deprived* of the traumatic experience[13] of mutilating himself in order not to disappear completely as a possible budding subject. The aim is to survive: to stay alive by staying connected to the scene—invested as original, not originary—of the failure of the helpful other. The (deprived) subject of the traumatic experience, by his willingness to assume the fault and the guilt, and to incorporate them, experiences a solitude synonymous with abandonment, is condemned to relational incapacity, to being dismissed as a subject, different, no longer belonging to the community of fellow human beings. This is the essence of traumatic solitude.

If, subsequently, the deprived subject threatened with erasure has the opportunity to engage in a relational experience in which the other brings about his own erasure as if it were a disappearance, and this time the subject can recognise what has occurred and assume at least partial responsibility afterwards, he may be able to transform his traumatic solitude, to some degree, into potentially creative solitude. That is, a solitude allowing him to communicate with his fellow men in their shared experience of expecting a helpful other.

This expectation, reawakened in every libidinally invested relation, always proves disappointing to some extent. The expectation of reducing the other to the function of the helpful other *cannot but be* a disappointment to some degree—part of the shared human experience of solitude encountered in any relationship. The aim of any relation, seen in this light, would be to transform expectation into hope. In the traumatic context discussed here, the entire difficulty lies in this: *hope has no reason to be.*

The traumatic experience, initially self-mutilation which inscribes in the subject the absence of the other—psychic self-mutilation as a *condition* for survival, a survival experienced as an unsurmountable obstacle to bringing oneself into the world—could subsequently become a creative potentiality in the service of life. This potentiality is what can bring about *making contact with* the other in the self, both in one's internal life and in relations with others. In other words, solitude can become lively and liveable: no longer the place where one is deprived of the other, but the foundation of the relation with the other.

Notes

1 This chapter reproduces and adapts to the focus of the present work the article "L'impossible question de la possibilité du pardon. À propos de Primo Levi," *Revue française de psychanalyse*, 80 (1), 2016: 149–161.

2 Levi, P., *The Black Hole of Auschwitz* (original Italian title: Asymmetry and Life), Polity, 2005.

3 Levi, P., *The Black Hole of Auschwitz* (original Italian title: Asymmetry and Life), Polity, 2005, p. 182.

4 This approach will be developed *infra*.

5 Zaltzman, N., *De la guérison psychanalytique* (On Psychoanalytic Recovery), PUF, 1998, pp. 14–17.

6 Zaltzman, N., *De la guérison psychanalytique* (On Psychoanalytic Recovery), PUF, 1998, p. 17.

7 Zaltzman, N., *De la guérison psychanalytique* (On Psychoanalytic Recovery), PUF, 1998, p. 16.

8 This perspective is based on that of Jankelevitch, V., *L'Imprescriptible*, Seuil, 1986.

9 Levi, P., "The Grey Zone," in *The Drowned and the Saved*, Vintage, 1989.

10 Levi, P., "The Grey Zone," in *The Drowned and the Saved*, Vintage, 1989.

11 Levi, P., *The Voice of Memory. Interviews 1961–1987*, Belpoliti, M. and Gordon, R. (Eds.), Polity, 2001.

12 Levi, P., *If This Is a Man*, Everyman's Library, 1999.

13 Deprived, even in danger of erasure as a subject, to the point of possibly being aspired by the disappearance.

Chapter 8

Writing against...[1]

"How wonderful it would have been had I been able to exchange views about all this with my mother, with Alice Miller,"[2] the last words of Martin Miller's autobiographical essay are very clear. *The True "Drama of the Gifted Child"* is a book written by a son about his mother, to take the place of an exchange between them which could not happen.

The object of the exchange that did not take place consists of the application to one "case," by the son who is now a therapist, of the three fundamental elements of Alice Miller's theory. The case is that of both the son and the mother—an indistinction inscribed in the reference to (absorption) of the mother's famous book title in the son's book title. These three elements are: the attention given to the "development of the true self"; the therapist as "lucid witness"; "the transformative power of biographical work." These elements constitute the three markers of maternal failure or mistreatment which Martin denounces.

This, then, is writing *against* the mother: staying as close as possible to her theory *and* protesting against its misuse where she and her son were concerned, and testifying to the good use he makes of it—for her, for himself, and as a therapist. The book protests against Alice Miller's misuse of her own theory, against a theory based on the author's maternal failure, which reduced the son to a necessary victim. This is the premise of the book and the question raised by Martin Miller.

The theory of the mistreated child, central to his mother's work, is presented by the author both as pivotal in his training as a therapist, and as lacking, for Alice Miller, a true foundation in clinical practice. In fact, he points out that her theory was constructed on her rejection of psychoanalysis and her abandonment of any clinical practice. Here, the contradiction stems from the status underlying the son's "biographical" writing: son and therapist. The author claims double legitimacy: as the mistreated son of his mother, on the one hand, who was first her silent victim and observer and later the "empathetic listener" who heard her elaborate her theories; and on the other hand, as a therapist who tested the relevance of these theories in his practice. The biographical essay literally takes the place left vacant by Alice Miller in terms of autobiographical writing as well as in the discourse addressed to her son.

DOI: 10.4324/9781003542483-11

A mistreated son writes the biography of his abusive mother, author of theories on the mistreated child. He reveals her past as a mistreated daughter, which she tried not to see and to hide from others, repressing it through her actions and later in her theorising. The scene is structurally phantasmatic, as if the son cannot ignore his desire to personify for his mother *the wise baby*,[3] which she lacked within herself and which she needed to found her theory. Or as if he cannot escape the desire to have his body recognised as the body absent from the theory of a mother whose mother's body is absent.

In effect, what is evident here is the desire—after the mother's death—to reveal at once the mistreated child his mother had been, and the one he had been: that is, the desire to make his mother recognise the reality of her own abuse, and thereby restore a mother's body to her, so as to give himself a son's body.

In 2010, a few weeks after Alice Miller's death, in an interview with a *Spiegel* reporter, Martin Miller used the term "personal tragedy"[4] to speak of the pain he suffered as a result of the failed communication between him and his parents. Four years later the subtitle of his book displaced the tragedy onto his mother's personal life: "The Tragedy of Alice Miller." Thus, the aim of the book would appear to be simply the designation of the "true" subject of the tragedy. But I feel something more radical is at stake: testimony in the aftermath about confrontation with the paradoxical violence of a disappearance to be embodied for someone who is not there. The book serves to make official the construction of a subject acting as a witness, who can ask: who does the body of the abused child *belong to*? The psychic separation involved here does not result simply from the work of mourning, to which the book testifies, but also from the survival of an original disappearance, to which the book also testifies in retrospect—a guarantee, or merely a promise, of thirdness.

***

Thus, the book offers a biographical reconstitution of Alice Miller's life, on which I need not comment. My remarks will concern instead a few significant elements of Martin's autobiographical reconstruction of his own life. As long as we keep in mind that we are dealing with a reconstruction, these elements are more useful for staying close to his point of view, which is the exclusive focus of my present discussion.[5]

Martin was born in 1950, when his parents were finishing their doctoral theses. From the first, he was rejected by his mother, upset by his refusal of the breast. At two weeks he was taken in by his aunt for six months. Later, when his sister with Down's syndrome was born in 1956, Martin was placed in a children's shelter for two years. He describes two unstable, cruel parents and a home where the atmosphere was always violent: his father alternated between showering him with attention and indulging in physical and verbal aggression, while his mother alternated between indifference and intrusive behaviour.

After working as a teacher, in 1980 Martin undertook to study psychology, followed by training leading to practice as a therapist. This was the only peaceful period in the relationship between mother and son, the latter describing himself as her primary interlocutor during this period of creative effervescence when her first books were being written. But Alice asked her son to undertake primal therapy and imposed an insane therapeutic modality which almost drove Martin to suicide: the therapist worked under supervision and sent her supervisor the recording of the sessions; the supervisor, in turn, reported their content to Alice Miller. Moreover, she tried to forbid her son from becoming a therapist, considering him dangerous for his patients and publicly disavowing his therapeutic practice—something he only learned later through third parties. This caused a more or less definitive break in their relations, lasting until Alice's death in 2010.

***

In a letter dating back to this period, quoted at the beginning of the book, Alice Miller *explains to her son what he should know* to release her from her responsibility and take it on himself. She draws a parallel between the abuse inflicted by her mother and that inflicted by her husband, in order to differentiate her refusal to identify with her abusive mother from her son's enacted identification with his abusive father. This identification with the abusive father, she claims, grants the son permission to treat his mother like a child who can be abused—something she owes it to herself to refuse *for his own good*—it is for your own good that I must condemn the abusive father in you by revealing the abused child you have turned me into. Here, the cruelly destructive innocence of good intentions reaches its apogee, in an incredible illustration of the "terrorism of suffering" that Ferenczi denounced.[6]

The mother presented here by the son is innocent, even going as far as recognising her failure to "save" her son—a son caught in a guilty act he is consequently asked to avow: a rejecting son, a bad patient, and a therapist to be rejected. The mother plays the role of therapist to escape the role of mother—the mother she had been, inadequate and hateful, as well as the mother she has not been: receptive and ambivalent—by illustrating with and against her son the solid basis of her theory of the abused child. This proves to confer a double benefit: it puts her in touch with the abused daughter she herself was, making her forget the abusive mother she was, and the fact that she constructed her theory after giving up the practice as a therapist. Here, we are at the very heart of the incestual confusion of places theorised by Ferenczi and taken up in large part by Alice Miller in her work. There is no room for Martin as a mistreated subject; he is disavowed as the subject of speech and as a witness, and prevented from providing his traumatic experience *as proof*.

In other words, not only must she occupy the place of therapist for her son, he must be theorised—terrorised?—so that she will not be the mother of an abused son, and thus avoid acknowledging her identification with, or even incorporation of, her own abusive mother. There is no room for two mistreated children: the abused child is solely her. The absence of her own body, the body of a mistreated child, in her writing about the abused child no doubt indicates her traumatic disappearance from herself for "sixty years"—a fact which also constitutes a denial of her hate for her mother, an unconscious sign of loyalty to their indissoluble bond.

In this letter, Alice Miller portrays herself as personifying entirely, consistently, and exclusively the abused child: by her parents, by her husband—chosen to reenact most closely her mother's cruel innocence—and finally by her son, who mistreats her without seeing that he attacks her just as his father attacked him.

By using such a letter as an epigraph, the son very likely wants to testify *to the fight to the death for life* which he had to wage *against* his mother and *with* her theory. It is in this light that we must evaluate the biography he wrote after his mother's death, and his Preface to a new collection of four of her most important works. In his own words: "As Alice Miller's son, I have followed from the start, and in a privileged way, the development of her thinking. Moreover, in the past thirty years while working as a therapist, I have also had occasion to apply her theories."[7]

He writes from the position of a survivor of his childhood—the childhood of a child of survivors—a position whose stated objective is the reconstitution of Alice's life during the Nazi period, about which her son had known almost nothing, as well as the reconstitution of the psychic effects of Nazi persecution on Alice Miller.

> Survivors want nothing more than to undo their experience. They erect a wall of silence and split off what they have experienced. They avoid any situation that reminds them of what they have been through. Unfortunately, they do not succeed; rather the next generation is woven into the split-off horror of those experiences and thus taken as hostages into captivity. This is my role in the persecution history of my mother.[8]

By writing his book, Martin Miller takes back the power to identify with his mother by freeing himself from the omnipotence she lays claim to as a bestower of identity. In this way, Martin retroactively recovers his identity as a surviving child, by ridding himself of the "inverse relation," the "parentification" imposed on the child by the splitting of the surviving parent. He reminds the reader that a survivor's child is required to adapt to the needs of an "emotional counterpart,"[9] which had been lacking for the parent. But Martin can't help justifying his mother's maternal "incapacity," blaming it on a consequence of the "the Nazi persecution of the Jews."[10]

What is at stake for him is crucial: to succeed in convincing himself that his mother's persecutory behaviour towards him was the result of the trauma caused by the Holocaust. But his certainty can only be based on denial, since at the same time he describes his mother's attitude towards him as having emerged in two stages: first at his birth, and later, in its persecutory form, when her son became a therapist, precisely when she had developed her theory of abuse and had given up clinical practice as a consequence of her rejection of psychoanalysis. But the precision of the biographical reconstitution—which never admits to being a reconstruction—does not do away with denial:

> Nevertheless—and this is very important to me—I do not see this book as yet another offering in the series of reckonings in which children of prominent personalities judge their deceased parents harshly. Nor do I intend to suggest that my mother's behavior toward me negates the merits of her books and the importance of her theories.[11]

The extenuating circumstances explaining the destructive split characteristic of having survived does not concern only the person who survived the Holocaust, but above all, the one who survived parental pathology. This applies particularly to maternal cruelty, mercilessly innocent, which inspired the idea of "poisonous pedagogy" in Alice Miller's second book *For Your Own Good.* From this perspective, the author presents his mother as a daughter forced to identify with her mother.[12]

The book can only partly be read as a reprisal for his mother's domination: after having been defined by his mother, Martin now describes his mother and their relation based on her theory. But the book does not want to be a "settling of the score." First, it expresses his wish to share the status of abused child with her, a wish left largely unrealised, but whose fulfilment would have put an end to repetition. Here, the question of the body in the act of writing is crucial.

Martin Miller's writing aspires to be the place where a son and a mother are reunited: a place free of hate and incestuosity, a place of reunion separating the bodies to make clear the similarity of their abuse by a rejecting and murderous mother, beyond the Holocaust and its transgenerational effects. The aim of the son's writing is to consecrate his mother's writing as a place where, for her, the body and the mind can be reunited, overcoming the dissociation in her own life between theoretician of the abused child and abusive mother. While the mother seems to claim that the theory does not annul the possibility of *not* being obliged to live, the son claims the theory as a place of existence for her—the theory or, more accurately, the thinking process underlying writing.[13]

The author wants not only to save his mother's theory but to prove that it can be *put into practice*, by testifying to the use to which he puts it in his own clinical practice. Given that he was deprived of a mother in his childhood, he turns himself into his mother's child by basing his clinical practice on her theory, which he questions at the same time. No doubt he did this at the cost of provoking melancholic reprisal in his confrontation with a mother who preferred deceased interlocutors to those still alive.[14]

The same personal motivation is what seems to drive Miller to apply his mother's theory to his clinical practice, and to think of it, in their relationship, both as having survived his mother's murder *and* her murderous mothering. This mother, killed and a killer, constructed herself and was kept alive by her hate for her parents, particularly her mother, a hateful and envious mother she had introjected—to survive her abuse and to prevent losing her. And hatred *of and for* the mother can only exert a conserving function through attachment to the body of the abused/

abandoned child, safeguarding the relation with the hateful/hated mother. In this perspective, the disassociation between theory and life could serve to safeguard the body of the hated/hateful child, literally isolated by the theory, submitted to a thought process instead of being experienced. As a result, the theory is projected on Martin.

It would appear that disavowal of her Jewish identity[15] helped Alice Miller survive Nazism, hide who she was and show a particularly creative adaptive capacity in the interest of survival, enabling her to take initiatives that saved the lives of her family members as well as her own. But no doubt this disavowal also allowed Alice Miller to remain identified with her mother, and, above all, *by* her mother, by continuing to be an abused child for whom splitting was a vital need. Recourse to splitting and mobilising hate in the service of survival was vital to Alice Miller, along with the denial of this hate in her self-destructive behaviour with her son.

Transference of the parent's hatred onto Judaism shows the great extent to which this adaptive creativity originates in the construction of a "false self"[16] in childhood. It was as if Alice Miller had erased—despite having internalised it—the relation between surviving Nazi persecution and surviving maternal persecution.[17] However, here too the book presents the author's mother as having been guided by her theory. The son explains that his mother reproduced with him the cold cruelty her mother had shown her.[18] But by saving his mother as a theoretician, by expounding on her theory as she applied it in her practice, he assumes, in spite of her, the role of a son ...[19]

He no doubt needed to make us witnesses to a crucial turning point, as catastrophic as it was lifesaving: his becoming a therapist. This necessarily set in motion the murderous mechanism the mother used to prescribe a therapy for her son, to supervise this therapy and then disqualify him as therapist—the only means he had found to survive and save their relation from her destructiveness. This was the murderous mechanism used by the mother to repeat the inaugural projective scene, which in fact takes the place of the son's originary scene: "From the beginning, you refused to feed at the breast. I was very offended."[20]

***

It appears likely that for Martin Miller his book creates a testimonial space which inserts an element of thirdness, in the aftermath, between him and his mother: *a text in his name*, writing through which he can be the son—albeit the abused son of an abusive mother who had been an abused daughter, but without being either her therapist or her patient.

Once he wrote this book, and now that he has conducted the necessary research using written documents and testimony he collected, Martin has no doubt freed himself from Alice's maternal hold. That is, freed himself from the position of "silent witness" that his mother tried to perpetuate indefinitely. Martin accomplishes this by recourse to Alice Miller's own terms—terms such as "enlightened witness" or "helping witness"—in the elaboration of the testimonial narrative presented in this book.

Notes

1 This chapter reproduces in a modified and augmented manner, suited to the perspective of this book, the analysis of Martin Miller's book presented in Chiantaretto, J.-F., "Présence et absence du corps dans l'écriture de soi: Martin Miller *contre* Alice Miller," in Chiantaretto, J.-F., and Matha, C. (Eds.), *Écriture de soi, écriture du corps*, Hermann, 2016, pp. 9–22.
2 Miller, M., *The True "Drama of the Gifted Child,"* independently published, 2018, p. 163.
3 The absence of any explicit mention of the Ferenczian concept of "wise baby," so obviously referenced by the author's discussion, can clearly be attributed to repression.
4 Miller, M., *The True "Drama of the Gifted Child,"* independently published, 2018, p. 163.
5 Miller, M., *The True "Drama of the Gifted Child,"* independently published, 2018, p. 163.
6 Ferenczi, S., "Confusion of Tongues Between Adults and the Child," *Contemporary Psychoanalysis*, 1988, 24: 196–206.
7 Miller, M., "Du côté de l'enfant—Une approche subversive de la souffrance humaine" (Preface), in *L'essentiel d'Alice Miller*, Flammarion, 2011, p. x.
8 Miller, M., *The True "Drama of the Gifted Child,"* independently published, 2018, p. 61.
9 Miller, M., *The True "Drama of the Gifted Child,"* independently published, 2018, p. 61.
10 Miller, M., *The True "Drama of the Gifted Child,"* independently published, 2018, p. 61.
11 Miller, M., *The True "Drama of the Gifted Child,"* independently published, 2018, p. 19.
12 Miller, M., *The True "Drama of the Gifted Child,"* independently published, 2018, p. 19.
13 Miller, M., *The True "Drama of the Gifted Child,"* independently published, 2018, p. 19.
14 Miller, M., *The True "Drama of the Gifted Child,"* independently published, 2018, p. 19.
15 The hate-filled relation to Judaism seems inseparable from the mother's relation to her parents, especially her mother. Objection to the fourth commandment of the Decalogue— "Honor your father and your mother, that your days may be long in the land which the Lord your God gives you"—holds a central place in Alice Miller's theory. Her limited knowledge of biblical texts is easy to see, but what is even clearer is the hate and anger aroused by what she sees as her family's religious alienation. At least according to her son, who allies himself with her, once again to *explain* her pathology through causality.
16 Miller, M., *The True "Drama of the Gifted Child,"* independently published, 2018, p. 19.
17 The author quotes from a letter written by his mother.
18 Miller, M., *The True "Drama of the Gifted Child,"* independently published, 2018, p. 19.
19 Miller, M., *The True "Drama of the Gifted Child,"* independently published, 2018, p. 19.
20 Miller, M., *The True "Drama of the Gifted Child,"* independently published, 2018, p. 118.

Part 4

Borderline Existence

The body as the dwelling place of life—the space of life, of the incarnation and acceptance of the gift of life—is also the inaugural place of psychic life. That is, the place where self-preservation, sensoriality, and autoeroticism meet, an encounter whose effectiveness and quality depend on what Ferenczi, before Winnicott, described as a good enough welcome provided by the environment. A good enough welcome means an arrival the *infans* experiences in his body as sufficiently gratifying to the primordial other, at the sexual and narcissistic levels—thanks to the partly reciprocal added pleasure springing from the satisfaction of his vital needs. Thus, the welcome provided by the narcissistic and sexual investments of the other who fulfils basic needs allows the infant to find/create his body as a welcome guest: the body welcomed by the psyche, the psyche welcomed by the body. In other words, after Ferenczi, autoeroticism is to be regarded as a merging of the body and the psyche, as a space and a register, as (self)representation and as the sphere where one's own and the other's narcissistic and sexual investments come together.

The representable body acts as a bridge between being alive and living, between the living body and the libidinal body. The body is rendered representable by the capacity to represent and invest itself, which determines the feeling of existence and continuity belonging to the narcissistic foundations of the being. Thus, autoeroticism can be seen as an unfolding of the body, an act of exploration prior to the emergence of the subject, his thought process and his objective: the embodied being. Autoerotic exploration creates the sexual by finding it, thanks to the other's narcissistic and sexual investment.

But how can this *investigative* capacity of the *infans* emerge when to live implies to partially forgo representation, the advent of a representing faculty, given the need to survive the discontinuity of the psychic presence[1] of the environment? Borderline existence is likely a consequence of having survived the pain of having had to live without durable assurance of surviving. One would have had to survive the pain of experiencing the satisfaction of one's vital needs by the other—to a degree sufficient to sustain life—without feeling oneself exist permanently and confidently enough in the other's investments, in the pleasure of being thought of with pleasure by the other.

DOI: 10.4324/9781003542483-12

In addition to the need to distinguish between the many forms of the border-line phenomenon,[2] borderline existence can be said to designate a survival mode consisting of self-investment in a relation to others which is seen as inevitably condemned to disappear from the other's thoughts. The subject of this existence is threatened with disappearance all his life; to bear the state of being alive, he condemns himself to imagine that he is already in the process of disappearing for the other.

Notes

1 A presence rendered deficient by the primordial other's absence to himself and to the other, to the point of possible disappearance.
2 Borderline psychopathology—the borderline register—imposes the use of a transnoso-graphic approach to the different types of psychic functioning involved to various degrees: from borderline problems undermining certain neurotic organisations, to outright borderline organisations, setting aside disagreements about their designation (borderline states, borderline functioning, etc.). I believe the borderline sphere delimited in this manner must be distinguished from all other forms of psychotic structuration; in this, I differ from other authors, and first of all from Harold Searles.

Chapter 9

Disappearance *or* Loss

What makes it possible to survive the first inscription in the infant's being of the discontinuity of the psychic presence of the other—this unliveable inscription with no possible representation? This is the question raised by so-called borderline patients. These patients have had to survive the subjectively experienced disappearance of the other; they desperately cling to this survival, renewing it endlessly in their present relationships with others. The vital need for self-representation can only become liveable for them through the analyst's openness to hate in the countertransference—liveable: the source and substance of the pleasure of seeing oneself be, sufficiently freed from self-destruction.

Winnicott's text[1] is inaugural in this respect, insofar as it presents a model of countertransference based on a theory of the infant's vital dependence, a theory which is a radical departure from Freud's conceptualisation. The analyst's countertransferential hatred, if he is able to process it as a reaction to the denied hatred of the analysand who is facing a re-emergence of the originary dependence, authorises the latter to feel his hatred in an altered form. He can then gain access to a hatred that separates, that can free itself of the predominantly narcissistic nature of his investments, which reduces the other to a subjective object. But the propositions made in 1947 do not suffice to arrive at a complete understanding of hate in borderline cases.

What makes living possible after having had to survive the state of absolute dependency and powerlessness unavoidable in infancy? This common fate—albeit not uniformly borne and not uniformly contributing to creativity, takes a radically paradoxical form in a borderline context: how is it possible to live differently than by having survived one's survival through self-destruction? Winnicott's last major paper, "Fear of Breakdown," makes it easier to consider the question, when we read Winnicott with Ferenczi in mind.

* * *

The analyst's hate is a reaction—a transformative reaction—to the self-hatred the borderline patient awakens in him: a self-hatred which undermines his very ability to invest himself in his work as an analyst, his ability to invest the patient as the

DOI: 10.4324/9781003542483-13

source of an unprecedented "thinkable," of *potentially mutual* narcissistic gratification, accompanied by a surplus of (auto)erotic pleasure for each of them. What draws the patient into the transference is his need to prove that any other is a disappointing helpful other,[2] and that he himself is unlovable by nature, condemned to be disappointed or disappointing—one or the other—forever. What is involved here is surviving the unfathomable disappointment experienced by the *infans*: being disappointing for the other on whom his life depends, and unable to feel the disappointment the other causes him—the other absent to himself when the *infans* needs his presence. Surviving requires investing oneself in one's ability to be disappointing, to the point of reducing oneself to a disappointing being: a disappointing being born of a disappointment imagined to be shared—a confusion that is literally vital, since this alone can render liveable—through denial or disavowal—the loss of self in the other who has become absent to himself.

If the hatred felt by the analyst can be transformed into hate towards the patient, the latter will be able to identify the true object of his own hate: the analyst's psychic presence to himself in his ability to take pleasure in the unfolding of the psychic presence of the other to himself. This attractive presence is totally intolerable to the borderline patient, because it promises what the *infans* expected and did not receive: to be included in the narcissistic and sexual investment of the first other.

This presence represents a paradoxical threat of disappearance because it opposes the mode of survival as a disappointing being, which made it possible, through self-effacement, to make an active investment in being condemned to disappear, and thus to save oneself and the other from disappearing to oneself. The process involved in this survival strategy—threatened by the analyst's investment and by the analyst himself—can be likened to a negative narcissistic identification, very close to an incorporation. The line between them is a narrow one: to identify with the denial the other inflicts on himself, and to invest oneself/invest him as one capable of disappearing or making disappear—perhaps always in the process of vanishing but not yet vanished.

With the objectivation/externalisation of hate, it becomes imperative for the analyst to survive self-destruction and the destructive transference induced in the analysand. To survive it, the analyst must recover the ability to conceive of the analysand as separate from himself: in the investment of hatred as the object of a reflection capable of self-investment and self-observation once again, and no longer in hateful self-investment against which his sole protection is hatred of thinking. As for the analysand, the analyst's transformative activity will prove to be essential for enabling him to leave behind this very particular mode of surviving through self-destruction carried out by displacing self-hatred onto the other. Paradoxically, the experience of having felt the hate of the other as a mode of investment paves the way for self-investment in the investigation as a space of *shared* disappointment (disappointed/disappointing), and to the possibility of contacting in his own mental functioning—not in the other's—the infant threatened with disappearance. The aim to be reached by a borderline patient, from this perspective, is to separate himself from the original mutualisation of the disappointment suffered by the infant. Ferenczi's interpretation of "Mourning and Melancholia" is valuable in this context.

> ... the melancholic suicide actually commits a double suicide. He kills himself (his critical ego) and also his beloved (ego), which has proved to be unworthy of him after he (the narcissistic ego) succeeded for a time in deceiving him (the critical ego)! The occasion for the illness was effected by the disappointment in other persons who served as models for the narcissistic ego and the devaluation of whom also reveals one's own worthlessness. Melancholia is thus a case of unfortunate (unworthy) falling in love with one's self.[3]

How can the analysand be helped to attain this detachment, to resist the temptation of killing himself rather than having to bear the threat of disappearing in the transference? In other words, how can he be helped to face the melancholic resurfacing of the original threat of *having been made to disappear*? What it takes is contact with the human, the experience of "rediscovering the resemblance with an animated human being."[4] What must be rediscovered is what the *infans* lost after having experienced its possibility: the psychic presence of the other—an identifying force *to encounter* in autoerotic investigation.

In truth, here, for the risk of suicide to be circumvented, the patient must discover — in the Winnicottian sense of the word—rather than rediscover. He must find it, but where? Not in the relationship with the analyst and his emphatic attitudes, real or supposed, but in what he—the patient—can imagine or perhaps feel regarding the manner in which the analyst found refuge in psychoanalysis to be alone and think through the incitement effected by borderline transference—incitement to self-effacement and to erasing the analysand from his thoughts.

It is vitally important for the analysand to be able to *imagine* the analyst's intimate relation to the remainder still active in him of the infant's expectation of a helpful other—an expectation transferred onto the analysis, in order to overcome the distress associated with the helplessness felt in the presence of the disappointing person mutualised in the transferential sphere. And the analyst has no choice than to overcome this distress as well, by dismantling it in the words of his internal interlocution, that is, by differentiating and recognising his own distress: that which comes from re-experiencing, through the analysand, early, unrepresentable states of disappointment, relived as a sense of being *disappointing*.

Indeed, we might suppose that these states would have been relived with his analysts, but borderline patients are particularly skilled at soliciting the analyst in the areas where resurfacing manifestations lack sufficient interpretation. In other words, in the places where these remnants have woven together the unanalysed material in the analyst and his analysands, to produce the invisible but transmissible cloth of a disappointment shared by them, which was likely to produce, as a last resort, an imaginary confusion between the unanalysed and the unanalysable.

Here, borderline structures force certain analysts to overcome their resistance to psychoanalysis—by returning to Freud, to a re-reading of the Freudian corpus recommended by Laplanche, and to yet another re-reading after the Ferenczian new start. Winnicott constitutes a representative figure here, precisely due to his reluctance to recognise his debt to Ferenczi.

* * *

> I have attempted to show that fear of breakdown can be a fear of a past event that has not yet been experienced. The need to experience it is equivalent to a need to remember in terms of the analysis of psychoneurotics.
>
> This idea can be applied to other allied fears, and I have mentioned the fear of death and the search for emptiness.[5]

This posthumous text, written at the end of his life, discloses the heart of Winnicott's thinking process and presents a final metapsychological reformulation. Perhaps more unequivocally than any of his other writings, this text illustrates his transnosographic perspective as applied to the exploration of the mental universe of borderline functioning—an exploration he essentially initiated. Fear of breakdown, related to "the individual's past experience" and to "environmental vagaries," and only explicitly present as such in certain patients, is nevertheless a "universal" phenomenon. Related to the infant's absolute state of dependence, in the analysis this fear can only express itself by a reactivation of dependence in the transference.

We are dealing with an "unthinkable state of affairs" that underlies a defence organisation, not with a failure in the organisation of a defence. While in the sphere of the neuroses castration anxiety lies at the foundation of the defences, the "more psychotic" phenomenon considered to be fundamental here is the threat of a breakdown of the ego organisation, demanding that the ego organize defences. But the state of dependence prevents the ego from organising "against environmental failure."

"The individual inherits a maturational process," but depends, in order to receive it, on "a facilitating environment," which has its own characteristics, adapted to the maturational process of the individual: holding develops into handling to which *object-presentation* is added; in terms of individual growth, these characteristics facilitate *integration* first and then *installation* (psychosomatic collusion), followed by the *object relation*. When the environment is deficient during the period of absolute dependence, before the me/not me differentiation, when the mother still fills the function of auxiliary other, the infant can experience *primitive agonies* which will activate archaic defences:

1. A return to an unintegrated state. (Defence: disintegration.)
2. Falling forever. (Defence: self-holding.)
3. ... failure of indwelling (installation in the soma.) (Defence: depersonalization.)

4. Loss of sense of real. (Defence: exploitation of primary narcissism, etc.)
5. Loss of capacity to relate to objects. (Defence: autistic states, relating only to self-phenomena.)
   And so on.[6]

From this perspective, Winnicott disagrees with seeing psychosis as a breakdown: psychosis is "a defence organization relative to a primitive agony, and it is usually successful (except when the facilitating environment has been not deficient but tantalizing ..."[7]

Winnicott states his main contention as follows: "... clinical fear of breakdown is *the fear of a breakdown that has already been experienced*. It is a fear of the original agony which caused the defence organization which the patient displays as an illness syndrome."[8] In other words, "*the breakdown has already been*," and it was, by nature, impossible to integrate; nor was it accessible to repression by the unconscious in Freudian terms, because the ego at the time was too immature "to gather all the phenomena into the area of personal omnipotence."[9] This means that a past experience only found negative inscription, and awaits being experienced and taking place, because it has not been integrated. It can only exist psychically for the patient in the future, in the form of fear of an expected breakdown.

... this thing of the past has not happened yet because the patient was not there for it to happen to.[10]

Breakdown experienced before the constitution of the ego is unthinkable because there is no place where it can be inscribed, and because it is caused by the unthinkable deficiency of an environment on which the *infans* is vitally dependent. Experienced without the ego, the event awaits being experienced by the ego. This can only happen if the past is reactivated by and in the transferential relation, provided it places the patient in contact with the original state of dependence. Reactivation proceeds from the analyst's blunders (mistakes and technical errors) which, if not excessive, can be integrated as countertransferential content allowing the patient to experience in the present (gradually and painfully) and to integrate into the ego, the original breakdown. But this means that both analysand *and* analyst consent to give up "psychoneurotic analysis" (pleasurable for both parties), and accept experiencing "the thing feared."

Winnicott proposes the fear of breakdown as a metapsychological model applicable to the fear of death, of emptiness and of non-existence. For instance, the fear of death can be thought of as a threat of annihilation which "happened to the patient but which the patient was not mature enough to experience."[11] Emptiness is not related to a trauma, but is rooted in an early experience of "nothing happening when something might profitably have happened."[12] This experience precedes the me/not-me distinction and the constitution of the self; as an experience of "personal non-existence, [it] is part of a defence." Nevertheless, this element can have a non-defensive dimension, since "only out of non-existence can existence start."[13]

The idea that the catastrophe projected into the future has already taken place is a novel, fundamental concept which definitively defines Winnicott's contribution, at once metapsychological and psychopathological. Winnicott's approach sheds light on the psychic construction of the *infans* before the constitution of the self (even before birth), when it is in a state of absolute dependence and non-separation from the environment. What is described is the process itself: the creation of the psyche as a containing envelope and a dwelling place. A separate psychic space does not exist yet; therefore, the deficient environment—which would be better described as a failure constituting a true threat of annihilation—can only be inscribed as an impairment in the process of creating the psyche. This impairment announces the advent of the catastrophe: the threat of breakdown henceforth activated by the psychic functioning itself.

The fear of breakdown provides a model for theorising—before going on to the sphere of repression examined by Freud—a means of defence anterior to the constitution of the ego. We must point out that Winnicott based his conceptualisation of the fear of breakdown on its manifestation in the transferential dynamics present in the analysis of an adult. Here again, Winnicott adopted a Ferenczian perspective. In *Confusion of Tongues Between Adults and the Child*, Ferenczi presents the analyst's blunder—his denial of his lack of psychic presence, a factor of traumatic repetition—as an occasion for the adult patient to re-establish contact with the deficiency of his early environment, which was also denied; of course, this possibility of contact depends on the analyst's elaboration of past events. For Winnicott, like for Ferenczi—as the passage entitled "Futility in Analysis" testifies—the metapsychological approach to early traumatic experiences is inseparable from a metapsychological approach to the analyst's frame of reference and psychic functioning.

* * *

Like Winnicott's last major text, Ferenczi's "testamentary" text on the confusion of tongues opened a new metapsychological perspective, after Freud. This perspective would later serve as the foundation of the concept of incestuality developed by Paul-Claude Racamier.[14] The incestual, incest without *visible* sexual abuse, can be defined as a "climate," a register of narcissistic abuse to which neither the abused nor the abuser lays claim—not an organisation, but a psychopathological *register* which, moreover, cannot be associated with an organisation as such. Further discussion of Racamier's approach to the intrapsychic, familial, and group aspects of the concept is best left for another occasion. My purpose here is to elucidate the usefulness of the new Ferenczian perspective for borderline psychopathology.

"Incestual" confusion is related to soul murder, that is, the incorporation of a psychic murder already perpetrated upon the primordial other in the state of absolute dependence: a disappearance inscribed with no possible representation in the construction of the psyche, exerting an ascendant hold over the subject and compelling him to enact "the denial of the self by the self."[15]

Ferenczi depicts the scene of a murder with oneself as the only murderer, una-ware of his deed. The *infans* is forced to submit to the narcissistic demands of the other, who has been crushed by a distress that cannot be imputed to a subject—narcissistic demands with no erotic or autoerotic character whatsoever. This other is terrorised, not only by the unthinkable suffering of having been killed without being there, but also by the need to kill someone who is not there but whom he has the power to bring to life in himself. The stage which would make it possible to collect and play with oedipal phantasies of murder and seduction will never be permanently constructed: the thought of murder will always require surviving the murder of thinking.

Ferenczi extended Freudian metapsychology by rethinking the concept of narcis-sism. The adolescent, and then the adult, cannot take responsibility for his psychic functioning, and thus find his unique place as a subject, a *de facto* and *ex-officio* member of the human species, unless the infant experienced his psychic function-ing as a source of gratification at once erotic and narcissistic for the other on whom his survival depends.[16] Only on this condition can the solitude characterising the desiring being be attained: a liveable and enlivening solitude. This concurs with the Winnicottian model. Being connected without communicating; the precondition for being able to be alone is the experience of being with the other who is present in his absence: the mother is there simply by being present to herself, separate from the *infans*, which authorises him to be there by simply being present to himself.

The infant can be alone with his *preoccupation* because the mother, while being there, can see to her own *preoccupation* alone. Here, Winnicott describes solitude at the heart of the mental process, made possible by the pleasure the mother takes in thinking alone in the presence of the infant separated from her, whom she thus experiences in advance as a separate subject, autonomous, having secret contact with his internal world. It is as if thinking presupposes the mutual experience of separation of the mother and the *infans*, a source of narcissistic gratification and sexual pleasure for both, in two separate spaces, present in si-lence, without words.

This can be likened to "the right to secrecy as a precondition for thinking," pos-ited by Piera Aulagnier, who theorised thinking based on the analytic situation. The mother must make possible the pleasure of separation for the sake of immersion in thinking, a pleasure at the root of a state of desire in the register of sexuality. "To discover that one can take pleasure in thinking and to think about one's pleasure is the necessary prerequisite to any thinking activity."[17] We must add that while the mother's pleasure in thinking is guaranteed, the *infans* must give this pleasure to himself. "The thinking process is first invested as a creation one owes to oneself."[18] This statement could serve as a definition of creativity from Winnicott's perspec-tive. Locating creativity within oneself, the experience of being inside one's own creativity—this is the secret which determines thinking.

* * *

It is precisely this placing of creativity within oneself—this creativity which is also an appropriation—that is perverted in the borderline sphere, where the subject only exists through expropriation—endlessly repeated by him—of his creativity; in other words, when the secret is excluded. The borderline subject[19] *supposes he knows* everything about himself, so that he can efficiently ignore his own murder by displacing it on another.

This comes about as a result of the erasure of the unspeakable in the mother's investment in the *infans*, that is, according to Aulagnier, of the unspeakable portion of the maternal spokesperson's interpretation. In Winnicott's language, this concerns the incommunicable aspect of the constitution and occupation of an indispensable inner resting-place free of all relational obligations. This inner resting-pace is made possible by the mother's mode of presence/absence, which dispenses her and the infant of the obligation of being fully present, and which inscribes the secret at the heart of the psychical construction: at the heart of the maternal anticipation of the speaking subject.

Notes

1 Winnicott, D., "Hate in the Counter-Transference," *International Journal of Psycho-Analysis*, 30, 1949: 69–74.
2 The possibility being equated with the fact.
3 Freud, S. and Ferenczi, S., *The Correspondence of Sigmund Freud and Sandor Ferenczi.1914–1919*, Vol 2, Harvard University Press, 1996 [1915]. Letter of 25 February 1915.
4 Fédida, P. *Des bienfaits de la dépression*, Odile Jacob, 2001.
5 Winnicott, D. W., "Fear of Breakdown," *International Review of Psycho-Analysis*, 1, 1974: 103–107.
6 Winnicott, D. W., "Fear of Breakdown," *International Review of Psycho-Analysis*, 1, 1974: 103–107.
7 Winnicott, D. W., "Fear of Breakdown," *International Review of Psycho-Analysis*, 1, 1974: 103–107.
8 Winnicott, D. W., "Fear of Breakdown," *International Review of Psycho-Analysis*, 1, 1974: 103–107.
9 Winnicott, D. W., "Fear of Breakdown," *International Review of Psycho-Analysis*, 1, 1974: 103–107.
10 Winnicott, D. W., "Fear of Breakdown," *International Review of Psycho-Analysis*, 1, 1974: 103–107.
11 Winnicott, D. W., "Fear of Breakdown," *International Review of Psycho-Analysis*, 1, 1974: 103–107.
12 Winnicott, D. W., "Fear of Breakdown," *International Review of Psycho-Analysis*, 1, 1974: 103–107.
13 Winnicott, D. W., "Fear of Breakdown," *International Review of Psycho-Analysis*, 1, 1974: 103–107.
14 See Racamier, P.-C., *L'Inceste et l'incestuel*, Paris: Éditions du Collège, 1995.
15 As formulated by François Perrier. See *supra*: Perrier, F., *La Chaussée d'Antin*, Albin Michel, 2008.
16 Ferenczi, S., "The Unwelcome Child and His Death Instinct," *International Journal of Psycho-Analysis*, 10, 1929: 125–129.

17 Aulagnier, P., *Un interprète en quête de sens*, (An Interpreter in Quest of Meaning), Ramsay, 1986.

18 Aulagnier, P., *Un interprète en quête de sens*, (An Interpreter in Quest of Meaning), Ramsay, 1986.

19 Keeping in mind, of course, that there can only be adult borderline functioning *stricto senso* in the aftermath of the questioning, at puberty, of the psychical construction of the *infans* and the child.

Chapter 10

From Culture to Treatment

Malaise in Transparency

In *Civilization and Its Discontents*, Freud remarks that cultural development cannot be counted on to bring peace at the individual nor the collective level. And he goes on to say:

> And [ethics] does in fact deal with a subject which can easily be recognized as the sorest spot in every civilization. Ethics is thus to be regarded as a therapeutic attempt—an endeavour to achieve by means of a command of the super-ego, something which has so far not been achieved by means of any other cultural activities.[1]

Thus, the superego has a therapeutic function, but it cannot be expected to treat the culture, considered the *shared space* of individual subjects, or to treat these subjects. In fact, the discontent in question cannot be treated, for it is lodged deep in the hearts of men: it is "the constitutional inclination of human beings to be aggressive towards one another." And, above all, the superegoic commandment "You shall love your neighbour as yourself" must take into account the two aspects of the constitutional component: "the human instinct of aggression and self-destruction."[2]

The aim is not just to treat, but treat with care: take care of life, of the human in each individual and for everyone's sake—that is, regulate or even transform this "human inclination," at least in the sense of finding the minimally destructive forms it can take. In fact, is it not the case that the superego carries out a guardian-of-life mission here, since the treatment is the place where the individual and the collective are brought together, albeit in infinitely variable modes, depending on personal configurations?

These modalities, from the most brutal to the most moderate, from the most silent to the most tumultuous, ultimately prompted Freud to reconsider the precedence of masochism over sadism—reversing their previous order—and to define destructiveness as resistance to self-destruction:

> Impeded aggressiveness seems to involve a grave injury. It really seems as if it is necessary for us to destroy some other thing or person in order not to destroy ourselves, in order to guard against the impulsion to self-destruction.[3]

DOI: 10.4324/9781003542483-14

This harsh reality and its even harsher implications force us to regard the collective destructiveness of the human race as resistance to individual self-destructiveness, and to regard individual self-destructiveness as resistance to collective destructivity, that is, to the collective self-destructiveness of the human race. But here Freud maintains a metapsychological perspective which makes it possible to reflect on the intrication of the individual and the collective, beyond the question of destructivity. Piera Aulagnier theorised this perspective when she formulated her concept of a narcissistic contract:[4] the human race exists only through each individual subject, who only exists through the place that the human collectivity assigns him, and which he agrees to make his own. Nathalie Zaltzman's concept of the work of culture (*Kulturarbeit*) is founded on the same perspective.[5]

Here, the work of culture is seen as a collective safeguard of individual narcissism, of a "minimal internalised certainty of existence for the other": an "initial narcissistic capital."[6] This promise constitutes a shared libidinal space where human beings exist for one another, where the human is guaranteed in and for each individual, where belonging to the human species is unconditional. Each person is entrusted with representing the human, each individual is included in the future of humanity in and for everyone. In other words, it is in and through the individual psyche that the work of culture is carried out, and it is in psychoanalytic treatment that this work is most visible, relied upon and tested in the patient's transferential demand and the analyst's transferential and countertransferential offer.

Testing the consistency of the sphere between the two protagonists, a sphere belonging neither solely to one nor solely to the other, or solely to both, makes it possible to test, *between* them, the common ground common to all. But this is not a factor or a condition characterising the treatment; it is a victory to be gained through psychical work which *humanises* instinctual demands and *singularises* cultural demands—it is a process which extends the territory of the ego. From this point of view, what the patient gains exceeds his person—the gains brought about by recognising instinctual and cultural demands, both on the side of destructiveness and creativity: that is, experiencing the pleasure of clear awareness of the internal and external worlds. This victory also belongs to the analyst, and potentially to everyone, in the confrontation with the unavoidable presence in each individual of the "impulsion to aggressiveness and self-destruction".

"Cultural superego": Freud's term defines the superego as an entity which enforces the work of culture, an agent seeking to establish the right balance between instinctual demands sacrificed in the interest of communal life, and cultural demands sacrificed for the sake of instinctual satisfaction. The objective is to dose most appropriately the subject's natural inclination to aggressivity and self-destruction. *To dose most appropriately*: in a way best suited to the unique, particular configuration of the individual subject, given his narcissistic and sexual constitution.

* * *

Today, undoubtedly more than ever, malaise in the culture enters the analytic space and probably renders the cultural stakes in each analysis more visible. In the seemingly unlimited aftermath of the Holocaust, there arises the threat of the erasure of the human in each individual, the threat of a potential reduction of the human being to mere actual presence, without ambiguity or opacity. As if "Never again!" could finally be turned into an aspiration for limitless visibility of beings and of the world, with no obstacles to transparency.

The threat is no doubt reinforced by the proliferation and multiplication of the forms of exposure of the intimate, which are now present in literature and the arts as a manner of providing information and testimony, and which are supported primarily by the new communication technologies with all their means of self-presentation: blogs, selfies, etc.

The overexposure of the intimate tends to destroy intimacy, facilitating the emergence of a representation of the individual based on a belief in the possibility of doing away with the gap between appearance and being, what is said and saying, and between speech and communication. This belief gives birth to a subject deprived of shared solitude, of an intimate knowledge of the difference between the self and self-representation. This poses a direct threat to the internal alterity of the self and of the other: the enigma of the presence/absence to oneself, posed by the other, considered to be the indissociably intrapsychic and cultural element providing the possibility of living together.

Today's ideal of transparency has become an injunction, a more and more limitless injunction in the service of a recusal—going as far as denial?—of any negativity. This ideal holds an increasingly dominant place in contemporary society. The recusal it requires is the main source of destructivity, targeting the subject indissociably in the intimacy of his subjectivity and in his status as a member of the human species, regardless of his other affiliations. The double sense of "transparency" (to transpire) is essential for grasping the paradoxicality of the notion of coming to light, which presupposes disappearance, leading to the confusion between being and appearing. The declared positivity of the injunction to be transparent—everything must be visible!—is invoked to deny anything which opposes it, that is, the negative and invisible aspect of everything that exists. This can lead to the supposedly ethical requirement of making the invisible disappear, so that what exists and what is visible are made to coincide at last.

Fortunately, there is resistance! It exists first of all in the work with patients treated face-to-face, in psychotherapies Pierre Fédida described as complicated or difficult analyses, most often presenting borderline characteristics. For instance, one such patient, having just pointed out, as he often did, how much he resembles his father, added: "My father was always nonexistent, he was completely transparent." Another patient had been hidden as a child during the war; his father was deported when the boy was born, and after the war his mother abandoned him several times. During our first session, he told me he has still not "found himself" and added: "I only feel I exist when I am not looking at you."

In the first case, the transparency referred to designates the invisibility of the father to himself, in the eyes of that particular son. It is the visible manifestation of the self-effacement of the other, to whom one has to identify to prevent his disappearance, and to be divested of the power to bring it about. By contrast, identification, close to incorporation, requires self-effacement, which averts the threat of disappearing by eroticizing the guilty play between sadism overtly turned against the self, and denied destructive aggressiveness—a play that remains tied to the obsessional character of unconscious feelings of guilt.

In the second case, the aim is to find oneself—a hidden self—in the *intransparency* offered by the other's gaze, which makes it possible to hide one's own gaze; that is, to hide in one's own gaze and therefore feel alive from the inside. What is sought is the experiencing of the aliveness of one's interiority, confirmed in the present interaction with *the other expected in the transference*, who can create solitude that enables the subject to survive the disappearance of the primordial other—a father who disappeared and whose disappearance continued to manifest itself in the successive self-effacement episodes of an abandoning mother.

The two registers are different: one involves melancholiform depression superimposed on predominantly obsessional functioning. The other relies on the work of melancholia to survive the disappearance of the primordial other, that is, the melancholic threat of one's own disappearance. But in both cases there is a discourse carried by a transferential address testifying to self-reflexivity at work. This self-reflexivity—serving to express suffering in one case, and to designate a place of absence in the other—is stable enough to withstand a directed discourse, that is, *misdirected* discourse.

Both patients consent to seek, in the analyst's transferential offer, a personal way of resisting the internal injunction to self-effacement. The difference between them shows very clearly that borderline psychopathology concerns more than borderline functioning. Neither of these situations involves this functioning, although both problems are undeniably of a borderline nature.

The discourse of these two patients, taken together, reflects what is essential here: borderline psychopathology raises the question of the metapsychological status of the diversity of the elements related to the libidinal *charge* of the "initial narcissistic capital," as Nathalie Zaltzman theorised it. We can also look at resistance to self-effacement, to which the two situations testify in different ways, as an act of resistance to the social injunction to transparency. This injunction is becoming a normative demand in our society, in the service of collective self-destructiveness.

* * *

Resistance to self-effacement: these two situations provide a different view of the paradoxical aspect of the transparency that contemporary society is aggressively promoting through recourse to new "techniques of the self," to use Foucault's term. As Mazarine Pingeot[7] points out, visibility and invisibility are at their peak, and at the peak of their interconnection, but transparency is what this interconnection *brings out*. The paradox can be expressed quite simply: today, society pushes each individual to claim the right to be seen, that is, not to remain transparent, while at the same time demanding the greatest transparency on the part of individuals. The private, the sphere of "having" as a territory to exhibit, is taking the place of the intimate, which is in the sphere of "being" and takes the form of a secret space, the space of the secret. Presentation takes precedence over representation, and the substitute or the pseudo seems to ensure the predominance of exteriority over the intimate—"extimacy", to be understood only partly as Lacan defined it in *The Ethics of Psychoanalysis*: the reversibility of exteriority and interiority in self-representation.

This paradox seems to have found what I would call a catastrophic solution: as Byung-Chul Han[8] puts it, today an exhibited face is replacing the human countenance. In other words, instead of looking and being looked at, we are seeing and being seen: we no longer see ourselves in the eyes of the other; instead, we expose ourselves. The "evidence" of the visible erases the play of seduction and desire, which relies on the misunderstandings and blunders born of ambivalence—misunderstandings and blunders which we might call mistakes, but which give desire a chance to awaken desire. Transparency is pornographic, well beyond sexual revelation and sexual deviation. Transparency promises to erase the secret, the enigma of the solitude inherent in the feeling of being alive, and in the sexual and narcissistic pleasure of which it consists: everything must be visible, that is, *presentable* in the here and now, with nothing held back.

Resolving the paradox: everything must be visible, *therefore* everything is visible. The injunction to transparency enacts this doctrine, which is an effect of discourse, but of a discourse not appearing to be discourse, in its recourse to the strength of evidence. In other words, is it not the case that, more than being ideological, transparency is peculiar to ideology? Indeed, the effectiveness of ideology is determined by its ability to have no other representation but itself, that is, present itself as transparent discourse, both to itself and to the world—discourse without a subject. Ideology imposes the unstated statement of a one and indivisible worldview, providing a complete explanation of a world rendered coherent in and by the reduction of its reality to the logic of an idea.[9]

Is it not by declaring itself transparent that any ideology is, by nature, totalising and, at least potentially, totalitarian?[10] In the case of the present injunction to transparency, this self-proclamation has been radically accomplished: the injunction not only makes transparency its content, but makes this content reducible to its container. Beyond its explicit discourse, this injunction encourages the disappearance of the pairs of opposites which not so long ago constituted the foundation of the symbolic order: horizontality *versus* verticality, symmetry *versus* asymmetry. By doing this, the injunction advocates and promises an entirely immanent world, erasing the dialectical divide between visible and invisible, information and critical knowledge, communication and speech, surveillance and responsibility, contract, and law, etc.

I believe this to be a denial or disavowal of the sign, as pragmatic linguistics defines it. The sign only functions through an oscillation between presence and absence, that is, between the "potential opacity" of its materiality and the "actual transparency" of the statement[10, 11]. And this oscillation determines the sign's power of representation, which implies self-reflexivity of the representation itself. This self-reflexivity of the representation, linguistically recognisable, was translated into psychoanalytic terms by Piera Aulagnier, for whom all psychical representation presupposes a representation of the representation—an idea coherent with Freud's notion of language as an expression of thinking.

Seen in this light, self-reflexivity constitutes the target of the injunction to transparency, and is itself to be considered a statement of transparency. Transparency takes for granted an individual with a private identity, indivisible and unalterable, contrary to the psychoanalytic approach which requires confrontation with the divided subject of an intimate, undivided and altered identity. Jean Starobinski has explained clearly Rousseau's precept of a mythical age of transparency, safeguarding the essential innocence of the self, which men must rediscover in another form after the eviction of the gods as the sole witnesses, and the fall into the "wickedness" of social relations.

> The old transparency came from the naïve presence of men under the eye of the gods; the new transparency is an inward condition, a matter of one's relation to oneself; it is in the clarity of one's view of oneself that allows Jean-Jacques to portray himself as he is.[12]

For Rousseau, the autobiographical act constitutes the fullest expression of his unwavering effort to stay true to himself. The search for lost innocence through detailed and exhaustive self-narration can achieve its aim, that is, save the author from guilt, if he can produce a transparent presentation of himself for the reader. This transparent self-presentation is the lure constituting what I called the credo underlying the autobiographical scene.[13] By autobiographical scene I mean the enactment of a self-engendering phantasy, with construction in writing of a representation passing itself off as a presentation, a representation promising the reader that he shall see the author-narrator as the latter sees himself.

A self-engendering phantasy requiring the other as a witness, an affirmation of identity and testimony to internal change, the autobiographical scene displays internal interlocution. It claims to show how the author-narrator sees himself as he speaks, how he is reflected in his words, which constitute the witness to whom the reader is invited to identify. In other words, autobiographical writing shows precisely what it denies—in the sense of disavowing—internal alterity, the irreducible gap between the self and self-representation; the structural connection of the speaker with his interlocutor, as well as that of speech with internal interlocution; and the gap between loss of self and presence to oneself in the words.

To use a simple formula, "there is no I without you and no self without I." While the autobiographical presentation of the self, with its transparency phantasy, attempts to *disavow* the opacity of the internal alterity showing it at work, the contemporary injunction to transparency advocates outright *denial*.

* * *

According to Nathalie Zaltzman, the creative convergence of the work in the analysis and the work of culture produces "at least a temporary retreat of repetition compulsion," and "instead of recourse to illness, psychical work elaborates and confronts that which it would otherwise have attempted to exclude from its sphere of investment."[14] The aim of this confrontation is to eliminate the coincidence of the self with its representation, that is, to avoid a degree of self-transparency that can sometimes culminate in melancholic disappearance.

Making this change requires experience with the unrepresentable, the inescapable human need to face the unknowable. This presupposes "a surplus investment" more closely resembling a transformation of investments than sublimation—a redirection of sexual drives. The subject acquires greater access to the thinkable as it applies to "the human impulsion to aggressiveness and self-destruction": he can enjoy his thoughts, including thinking about self-destructiveness which negates thought.

> Eros cannot eliminate Thanatos ... Eros can only invest. But when it invests failures, impasses, ignorance of individual and collective history with new libidinal elements, Eros and the repletion compulsion force reason away from that which overwhelms it and which is found on the side of unreason, madness and murder.[15]

This alliance of Eros with the repetition compulsion, founded on a principle Zaltzman calls the anarchistic drive, could designate the refusal of transparency imposed by the work of culture in the analysis—as long as the strangeness of a shared solitude is facilitated—what Fédida would call the *condition* of the intimately strange. The intimately strange is the experience of the intersection of the stranger in oneself and the stranger in the other, in the encounter between the internal alterity belonging to each of them and the transference each makes possible for the other through his own transference and countertransference.

This absence of transparency is to be achieved by resisting the temptation of the familiarity of narration, a temptation present on both sides—one's own and the other's—to protect against the *Unheimlich* present in language. This victory is even harder to gain in complicated or difficult analyses—especially in face-to-face sessions—which tend to reduce discourse to a narrative, and the infantile past to the transferential present. In these cases, self-representation imposes a double constraint—transparency and communication—in order to refute any distance between the analyst to whom the transference is addressed and the analyst who hears the narrative, that is, the distance between speech and what is said.

This can result in a compulsion to say everything in an attempt to exhaust the transference, to empty the transferential space of its secret, the only secret in an analysis—and, in fact, its essence. We might think that in this type of case the analyst could tend to overinvest interpretation, paradoxically, as resistance to the transparency of a knowledge possibly shareable with the patient, a patient just as transparent to himself as he is to the analyst. Here, from a Winnicottian perspective, the role of interpretation is to force the patient and the analyst to realise that the latter does not know, that he interprets inaccurately. This would be a way to reintroduce nontransparent transference as a secret space.

As Nathalie Zaltzman wrote, the right to secrecy is the equivalent of the analyst's ethical and methodological commitment to refrain from taking advantage of the "position of power and abuse of power attributed to him by the patient"— attributed because the latter has already experienced it to some degree.[16] Respecting that which is unspeakable for the patient is a prerequisite for analysis; it is essential with psychotic patients, given that the unspeakable concerns the transgression of an injunction to death or to murder, enacted through the conception and birth of the subject—what Zaltzman called the "crime of lèse-Thanatos."

With non-psychotic patients, the prerequisite concerns the fundamental rule, which—most importantly in this context—corresponds to an invitation, not to *say everything*, but to say, *as much as possible, what comes to mind, just as it comes*.

Psychoanalytic thinking has its roots in the submission of the infant's and later the child's thought process to what the mother says. This involves an erasure of the secret investment of the infant by the mother, the source and condition of thought. Here, the thought process itself is attacked, while in borderline psychopathology what is attacked first is the self-representation of the subject in the process of thinking, even if the subject declares believing it to be possible, necessary and desirable to tell everything—a belief which will constitute his particular mode of resistance, if he is able to undertake an analysis.

In *An Autobiographical Study*, Freud pointed out that "the precondition of analytic treatment" consists of "the demand for candour on the part of the patient."[17] It is important to understand what this "candour" involves: it is the effort to find the words most closely expressing the inner experience to be conveyed to the other, while being present to oneself and to the other, in his presence. This is the opposite of a declaration of sincerity or of the impression of being sincere, which imply belief in the possibility of a coincidence of the self with oneself, of complete self-representation. This certainty of *being oneself*—the antithesis of psychoanalysis—must be clearly differentiated from the certainty of *being*, which underlies the feeling of being alive. The certainty of being oneself, which in neurosis always refers more or less directly to a self-engendering phantasy, can be seen as resistance literally offered to the analyst, as part of the transferential demand made to one who is presumed to know. In a context of neurosis, the patient addresses his demand at once, in good faith.

In borderline psychopathology—which also differs from a context of psychosis— certainty is focused elsewhere: the patient invests himself endlessly as the *victim of incest*, who knows what happened to him. He agrees to limit himself to the knowledge he presumes he has about what the other did to him unknowingly. Thus, he reduces any relation to yet another occasion to confirm his knowledge of being invaded by the unknown of the other: an imaginary knowledge, diverting or even blocking access to knowledge. As the sole possessor of knowledge which must remain out of the reach of anyone but him, and to which he can't help but block his own access—to avoid the risk of disappearing as a result of the incorporation of the disappearance of the other—the patient condemns himself to being an intruder forever.

In the borderline sphere, only certainty offers a remedy for the uncertainty related to the representation of one's conception and birth, made weightier by belief in one's definitive undesirable status—an unalterable belief in accordance with the principle of survival. Therefore, the patient tries desperately to lock anxiety away in the core of his being: there cannot and must not be room for "the anguish for being in the world."[18] And a compulsion not to know induces the thinking process, which claims to guarantee certainty by being the exclusive source of its production, to recuse itself.

The borderline patient does not offer the analyst his resistance. Transference is dominated by hatred, particularly hatred of the analyst's thought: a hatred which is naturally minimally or not at all representable. The analytic process can only proceed from the pleasure the analyst will take—despite and through his own hatred, the only possible response to, and representation of, the patient's hatred—in investing the investigation of the patient's psyche as a source of the questioning of his own psychic process. The difficulty for the patient, and consequently for the analyst, lies in this: in the borderline sphere, to be thought of with pleasure is an unimaginable pleasure because it can confer a sense of the unthinkable nature of the transferential demand—the unthinkable nature of love.

What is unthinkable is not the possibility of being loved, but that of being lovable. The patient has learned to survive with the certainty of being unwelcome, as Ferenczi uses this term in "The Unwelcome Child and His Death-Instinct." Indeed, by reactivating the infant's state of total dependency, the borderline transferential demand awakens in the patient the trusting expectation of the "exclusive other,"[19] an expectation emerging at the very site of the disappearance of the other, that is, at the place where the borderline subject has been condemned to live all relations with another human being as a promise of obliteration. For the subject's expectation, always renewed and always disavowed, that the psychic presence of the other has been acquired once and for all, while the denial of death is never certain, inevitably brings back the initial experience of disappearing in the disappearance of the other to himself, without a witness.

* * *

Borderline existence can be described as the obligation to efface oneself so as not to disappear *once and for all*, so as not to carry out against oneself, irrevocably, the other's disappearance to himself, experienced and internalised long ago,[20] when his vital needs made the *infans* totally dependent. The self-effacement of the other on whom his life depended has acquired the value of a disappearance for the subject of borderline existence—a subject in a state of perdition, always already lost, but always still to be lost in his relation with the other. Having to repeat this disappearance, both of himself and of the other, safeguards the subject by preserving as an inexpressible hope, the lost gaze of recognition that was, nevertheless, originally bestowed upon him. The expectation is to finally make perceptible an unformulable statement: *I have been disappeared.* An unbearable hope results from this—the possibility of an interpretation, the possibility that there could finally be a witness to this disappearance into the disappearance of the other.[21]

Being a source of pleasure in the analyst's thought process exposes the borderline patient to the danger of serious melancholiform depression, potentially apt to lead to a suicidal act. But only in this way can he advance towards *good* disquiet, the uneasiness that makes it possible to live with his fellow-men, consenting to difference *and* likeness, to repression of the past and to death as inherent to life.

Good disquiet is very different than the threat of disappearance in loss and absence. Good disquiet refers to the sharable disquiet related to being alive, existing in the singular solitude of each being, and accepting the enigma of incarnation and the gift of life. It also means the disquiet associated with the guilt of having to accept responsibility for one's functioning, having to bear being irresistibly and invisibly animated by what one cannot know about one's own desire, about the sources and motives of one's inclination to love or to hate. Ultimately, this disquiet is connected to giving up the innocence promised by transparency: consenting to be lost in order to be and feel oneself alive, consenting to the presence of death in life and beyond.

> Fear entered
> the body of the father who waits for his son,
> just as it entered, one day, the body of things.
> It was yesterday, it is today.
> It will be so even more tomorrow: the fear of the species,
> of species and of the Earth we thought so serene,
> but which keeps showing
> an angry countenance,
> as if it feels offended
> or is ready to revolt.[22]

Notes

1 Freud, S., *Civilization and Its Discontents*, S.E. 21, Hogarth.
2 Freud, S., *Civilization and Its Discontents*, S.E. 21, Hogarth
3 Freud, S., *Civilization and Its Discontents*, S.E. 21, London: Hogarth.
4 Aulagnier, P., *The Violence of Interpretation*, Routledge, 2001.
5 Zaltzman, N., *De la guérison psychanalytique* (On Psychoanalytic Recovery), PUF, 1998, p. 17.

6 Freud, S., *New Introductory Lectures on Psycho-Analysis*, S.E. 22, London: Hogarth.
7 Pingeot, M., *La Dictature de la transparence*, Robert Laffont, 2016.
8 Han, B.-C., *The Transparency Society*, Butler, E. (Trans.), Stanford University Press, 2015.
9 See Hannah Arendt, "Totalitarianism," in *The Origins of Totalitarianism*, Meridian Books, 1962.
10 In the sense of the attainment of a single goal.
11 See Recanati, F., *Truth-Conditional Pragmatics*, Oxford University Press, 2011.
12 Starobinski, J., *Jean-Jacques Rousseau: Transparency and Obstruction*, University of Chicago Press, 1988.
13 Chiantaretto, J.-F., *De l'acte autobiographique*, Champ Vallon Éditions, 1998.
14 Zaltzman, N., "De surcroît...? Le travail de culture? La guérison? L'analyse elle-même?," in Green, A. (Ed.), *Le Travail psychanalytique*, PUF, 2003.
15 Zaltzman, N., "De surcroît...? Le travail de culture? La guérison? L'analyse elle-même?," in Green, A. (Ed.), *Le Travail psychanalytique*, PUF, 2003.
16 Zaltzman, N., "Le secret oblige," in Aulagnier, P. et al., *La pensée interdite*, PUF, 2009, p. 51. It was the author's last conference, delivered a few days before her death on 11 February 2009.
17 Freud, S., *An Autobiographical Study*, S.E. 20, Hogarth, p. 40.
18 De Toledo, C., *L'inquiétude d'être au monde*, Verdier, 2010.
19 Fédida, P., *Des bienfaits de la dépression*, Odile Jacob, 2001, Chapter VII.
20 Here, internalisation can be equated with incorporation.
21 Etymologically, impossible to carry.
22 De Toledo, C., *L'inquiétude d'être au monde*, Verdier, 2010.

The Analyst's Transference, Transferential Writing

And for whom will I write then?

First Scene

A 10-year-old boy sees his father stab his mother to death in front of him. He is placed in a residential home and is assigned to the care of a psychologist he seems to like. After a few months, his work with the psychologist is interrupted when he is placed in a foster home. The referring educator suggests to the boy that he could see a psychoanalyst, if he agrees. At the first meeting, before the child arrives, she tells the analyst what happened to him, and mentions the boy's sleep and concentration difficulties, as well as his overwhelming sadness, which had prompted her to suggest a meeting with the analyst. Once the boy is with them, she emphasises his need to speak of everything that happened to him; the child smiles.

He continued to smile during the first two sessions, while he talked about his foster family and then drew in silence. He was drawing the scene of his mother's murder, and another family scene, apparently "normal," but with no father present. The analyst was disturbed because he was no longer certain of the murder scene as described by the educator, and he felt trapped in a position where he could neither *ask* the child to clarify, nor abstain from asking anything. Next, the child tore up the drawing of the murder, after which he fell resolutely silent, confronting the analyst with a provocative look, as if to say: "What is it? Why are you looking at me like that?" The silent interval was followed by even more provocative behaviour, testing the limits without great insistence, making a show of aggressiveness rather than acting it out.

As the sessions continued, brief moments of shared humour emerged, to accompany the provocation. Such moments occurred after two sessions where fright drove the boy to tears after an intervention made by the analyst in order to set certain limits the child was not to exceed. In this process, the boy's obsessive worry about the reliability of the analyst's promise not to reveal the content of the sessions (to the educator or the social worker) gradually faded.

In the first months of psychotherapy, the transferential role attributed to the analyst is that of a father who takes precedence over the mother (the psychologist or the educator), and who has the power not only to abandon (*planter*, in French) her, but above all to abandon the son, the witness to the murder, who has come to testify. The French word "*planter*" is to be understood in all three of its meanings: to stab, to plant, to abandon. The transferential figure of the father combines murder, conception and abandonment—fear of being murdered, quest for love and threat of loss. Thus, the analyst can assess at once the need for his (counter)transferential offer: the *reception* of the child's vital need to be heard, that is, to be invested more for what he offers than for what he asks, to be lovable for himself, since it is *for* the other that he is loved.

Second Scene

A man leaves a woman, the mother of his children. He leaves her for another woman, who has children of her own. With his wife, he liked to see himself as a survivor, and he loved her for her ability to survive their self-destructiveness. At that time, he placed the analyst in the role of a helpless witness forbidden to listen, kept in the position of an omnipotent mother who threatens a marriage bond founded on libidinal investment in a shared mode of thinking. With the second woman, he took the risk of loving and allowing love to survive *his* self-destructiveness, which he could finally acknowledge and test in his transference on the analyst. Now, the analyst is permitted to hold the position of a third party, a guarantor of the frame, and a father who can be killed—susceptible to be killed because he is alive: that is, able to survive hatred.

With his wife, the man, whose interiority did not enclose an other who loved him, was trying to make himself lovable as a depressed and unwelcome child. By doing this, he escaped his depression through recourse to action. This action aimed at displacing the hatred onto his wife, especially when she became a mother—his was a self-destructive hatred of the pathological femininity in both his parents. With the second woman, who would not tolerate his unloved child posturing, he tended to take a kinder attitude to himself by becoming aware of the depressed child inside him. He seemed able to desire and be desired sufficiently by the woman in the mother and the mother in the woman, while unmistakably playing—to please her and apparently to just the right extent—the phantasmatic role she required of him: a combination of the maternal and paternal figures.

To arrive at this result, the analyst had to submit for a long time to the workings of countertransference, which allowed the emergence in the transference of a hybrid figure with the combined fate resulting from the bad reception given to the feminine in both his parents: the figure of someone incapable of welcoming, that is, of nurturing; and equally incapable of separating, that is, of thinking.

Third Scene

A woman meets a man who leaves his wife for her. She has just started an analysis and would, for a long time, be obsessed with a phantasy: that the analyst sent this man to her as a sort of assistant, to help her to live and to carry out her analysis. She quickly moves in with this man—who has been in analysis for several years as well—and they undertake a sort of mutual analysis. In this undertaking, resistance manifests itself strongly: this "work" is reported to the analyst in detail; he is asked not only to approve of it, but to validate it in order to save the couple, which has been in trouble almost from the start.

Thus, for over a year the analyst is placed in a position where he has to stand by silently, watching the undoing of their relation. When the woman is finally able to start examining her feelings for the man, the analyst performs a countertransferential act: to reassure her, he asserts that she loves her partner. Now, she can start to hate the analyst and, consequently, truly start her analysis.

What the analyst did revealed to him his repressed hatred towards this patient who demoted him from his position, to replace him with her lover. In response, the analyst authorised the patient to express her hatred verbally, instead of acting on it—her hatred for the analyst, who defended her partner as a projective gesture, thereby protecting himself from both his hatred and hers. Her hatred was also directed towards her partner who, by playing the role of analyst, exerted a hold over her that was reinforced by her need for it, as it protected her from the risk of loving. The beginning of the analysis concealed and revealed the costly remedy used against the fear of losing love: hatred for the other in the face of an inability to love, a hatred serving to disavow the need for love that underlies desire. Confronting the fear of loss required clarifying the confusion between analysis and life.

Fourth Scene

A man lost his wife and his sister within a short period of time. Both died of aggressive forms of cancer. For many years he remained faithful to his deceased wife, taking care of his children in a house that remained absolutely unchanged. When he met another woman and established a stable romantic relationship with her, he experienced bouts of extreme bodily distress which prompted him to see an analyst. He had already seen other analysts at different times in his life, without ever being able to "use" them, in the Winnicottian sense of the word.

His fears, not of an outright hypochondriacal origin, manifested themselves solely in the abdomen and were related exclusively to his current love relationship. After a serious somatic attack which required emergency surgery, the fears surprisingly subsided and loyalty to his dead wife began to be seen as a protective screen against a strongly phallic mother, impossible to lose and just as impossible to love, who played the role of murderous mistress and killer of a father who had died long ago of a serious illness.

A few months later the mother died and the son sold the house he had shared with his wife. He went to live with his new partner in the city where he grew up, about 50 kilometres from his childhood home, in which his mother had lived. He decided to keep the house and use it as a family vacation home where his children and grandchildren could stay. Thus, the psychotherapy was interrupted after two years; but the patient's fears quickly returned. He telephoned the analyst, who had offered him this possibility. After two sessions by telephone, the patient took advantage of a trip to request a meeting in the analyst's office. This session turned out to be exceptional, in all senses of the word.

This session marked the return of the writer—the man was a well-known writer who made a comfortable living through the practice of his art. Now, what he was saying brought together for the first time, in a startling manner, two apparently unrelated elements. To start with, he noted an evolution in his writing, which changed from what he called "a family saga" focused on the paternal line, to purely fictional writing. In addition, he had started to express in writing, as he had never done before, his distressing bodily symptoms, concentrated in his abdomen: "a gap," like "a zipper that opens."

The catastrophe, which had found its place of inscription in the body, could finally be given expression in the words emerging in transference. Now the man's discourse lets the aftermath be enacted: after the mother's death, after the sale of the house (a separation from his deceased wife), and after separation from the analyst. This was confirmed in what he said about his writing, which was now freed from its previous mission: to relate the father's family story to the mother. When the psychotherapy was interrupted, words became capable of expressing anguish, including the anguish of the body; they were able to establish transference with the body.

It was as if the fact of having left an enigma with an analyst who consented to being left behind—without absenting himself in retaliation, without being driven to self-effacement by narcissistic vengeance—had opened onto the possibility of analysis elsewhere ...

At the end of this very special session, the man asked if he could come back for occasional sessions, scheduled to fit in with trips he was going to take, and the analyst consented. But in fact, instead of this arrangement, the man called the analyst to ask for the name of another analyst living closer to his new place of residence. A few months later, the analyst received a thank-you message informing him that analysis with the person he recommended had started.

Addendum

The Self in Question

Since I became interested in self-writing in all its forms, I have always thought that they must be defined by what they have in common, and which differentiates them from all other writing.[1] These forms of writing represent a certain mode of investing the act of writing, within the structure of a device founded on the narcissistic appropriation of words, making it possible to feel oneself exist under the gaze of the other. In other words, the device is dual: its nature can be indifferently scopic or linguistic. Its author himself describes it as a space of investment *for oneself and by the other*.

Setting aside subjective particularities such as literary genre and style, this device presumes sufficient confidence in the power of the words used in self-presentation: a true disposition to reveal oneself in words. This requires taking the risk—acknowledged and/or denied, knowingly and/or unknowingly—of revealing what one does not see in oneself, going as far as the invisible, as far as searching for oneself *to distraction* in the gaze of the other, in the hope or with the expectation of finding oneself.

This form of writing intends to present someone with someone else's interior scene: *this is how I see myself*. The authenticity of the scene is certified by the author himself, and requires certification by the reader, who is asked to adopt the viewpoint of the writing, as it is presented in the written text. Thus, writing is invested as the place of an internal experience of oneself in the words, supposedly expressed as such, in the *supposed* presence of the other, that is, calling as a witness a person who is absent.

This very particular recourse to the power of writing to create an illusion has helped me in my clinical work to understand certain difficult modes of being in which the absence of the gaze of the other, possibly announcing a disappearance, threatens to announce the disappearance of the self to oneself: *the loss of self*. For certain individuals, language fails—more or less seriously—to support and carry forth, to present and represent, to guarantee self-reflection, and to make it possible to see oneself thinking and being.

Once the hypothesis of the internal witness[2] has been accepted, experiencing oneself in writing, as well as the loss of self that threatens certain patients, both allow the investigation of borderline psychopathology. Here, the works of authors writing as Holocaust survivors[3] were decisive for me, not inasmuch as they testify to traumatic experiences and survival, but because they emerge out of the internal experience of loss of self.

This investigation follows upon the idea of a clinical practice enhanced by *an approach* that includes literary works, keeping in mind their irreducible nature and their necessary resistance to psychoanalytic interpretation, even when the text is a self-presentation of the author—a frequent occurrence in self-writing.

Although an analysand is not a text, and a text is not a pre-text for interpretation,[4] even and perhaps especially as regards self-writing, the irreducible question concerning what is interpretable when interpretation is carried out is, in both cases, the *path* the analyst must follow. The idea of a clinical practice enhanced by the reading of literary texts implies that the reading is inspired by experience with interpretation acquired in one's practice as an analyst.

Resistance to interpretation is the promise and the condition of the process of interpretive thought. This resistance is offered by what the text holds back. The interpretive process is potentially novel after each reading, potentially at the service of any reader's experience of transference, and potentially a source of creative thinking for the reader-analyst, elsewhere, in the transferential space shared by the two participants in the analytic session. The objective would be to receive the thinking presented in the works of writers,[5] rather than to apply psychoanalysis to literature. This work involves an irreproducible portion of psychical experience, which cannot be displaced without being altered. In other words, the thinking in literary works must evade any *external* fragmentary attempt at interpretation, because this thinking offers a *thinkable* sphere indefinitely widened by each reader's transference.

Nevertheless, the work of thinking proposed by the literary text is likely to help psychoanalysts think like psychoanalysts, provided they respect the specificity of such a text and, therefore, acknowledge the impossibility of translating it and displacing it, in order to place it as it is in the service of psychoanalytic investigation. *Helping the psychoanalyst to think*: when psychoanalytic theory is insufficient—based on his own experience with the psyche in the therapy and its variants—to think through the unprecedented aspect of the unthinkable revealed in each transference; in the place where, in the aftermath, his own recourse to writing will be enacted, in its intimate relation to the treatment; and finally in the place where writing can contribute on a metapsychological level to structure the space and the dynamics of the treatment, completing the contribution of dreams.

* * *

Aside from the "literary" foundations of Freudian metapsychology (Sophocles, Shakespeare ...), and even aside from the original transference onto writing in the first person, here Freud's oeuvre confronts us with his "auto-biography," that is, the position of self-representation taken in *The History of the Psychoanalytic Movement*, and in *An Autobiographical Study*. Both texts present the setting forth in writing the origins of psychoanalysis, a feat which carries out Freud's phantasy of being the sole witness to the conception of psychoanalysis, in himself as well as in his absence.

Thus, setting down the origins in writing constitutes an originary scene. Psychoanalysts are invited phantasmatically to see Freud's *conception*[6] through his eyes, to see the invisible through Freud's absence to himself while he strives to make the invisible visible. In this light, Freudian self-representation reveals the original strangeness of psychoanalysis to itself, a strangeness passed down to each analyst, who goes on to test it over and over in the strangeness of each transference. In addition, these two texts present a virtual model for a psychoanalytic approach to self-writing as self-presentation. The latter combines confirmation of identity *with* testimony of an alteration, and the enactment of a phantasy of self-conception *with* recourse to the other as a witness guaranteeing an identificatory mode of listening. This model renders reference to literary genres unnecessary, using instead an approach based on the specificity of phantasmatic aims connected neither with the author nor with a style or a genre, but rather with a reading pact suggested by the text. This mode of reading explicitly promises a self-presentation of the author himself, whose authority is certified by the declaration of identity connecting the author himself with the literary figures of author, narrator and main character.[7]

Thanks to its use of the modalities through which words enable a subject to see himself, self-writing presents not only an internal scene, but also a perspective. This perspective, constructed by the text as much as it contributes to its construction, shapes the belief of the author: to blend the self with self-writing, to look at oneself and see oneself in the eyes of the other. Belief in the total readability of the self, reliance on the other's gaze as if it were one's own, paradoxically exposes the subject to experiencing his own invisibility to himself and to the other.

In other words, the attempt to prove by means of writing the belief that one is oneself reveals the irreducible nature of internal alterity, indissociably in oneself and in the other: the strange stranger, with his power to modify a one-and-indivisible identity. Thus, the paradoxical nature of self-writing is enlightening for the analyst, who is confronted in the analysis with many transformations in the patient's belief of what it is to be himself. In this regard, the analytic work would consist of preserving and/or producing invisibility, that is, the strangeness of the stranger, a task accomplished variously—depending on the initial mission assigned to the transference—through repression, disavowal, or denial.

Someone sees himself reflected in the words, while seeing himself seen by the other, supposedly gathering together the others in himself—the internal voices of identification—and the potential totality of readers. The truth of self-writing does not lie in the content concerning events, relationships, and affective aspects of self-presentation; neither does it lie in content coherence and unity. This type of writing naturally supports the illusion of a unified version of self-representation, even when it is achieved by means of the most complex forms of deconstruction.[8]

The truth is more closely related to the internal point of view upholding the author's *I*. The paradox inherent to self-writing consists in the fact that this dimension of the truth is only accessible to the reader if he shares with the author the (illusory) belief that it could be possible to hold the place of the other in oneself—an *indivisible* place. Here, the other in oneself represents and suggests all the others distinct from oneself who donated identity, in the form of identificatory support, at all stages of life. Therefore, the term designates an ensemble of indefinitely multiple figures constituting an *identifying* viewpoint, an internal guarantor of the status of a fellow human being different from oneself: the internal witness.

The pact with the reader promises to show the author as he sees himself. It cannot keep this promise *in truth*, but gives the reader something else: the possibility of imagining what the author does not see about himself, and which drives him— that is, the manner in which his words bespeak him when he speaks to himself. And if the alluring promise is convincing enough, the text may make accessible—*in truth*, but partially and as an aside—the modalities of the close encounter between the author and the strangeness of the stranger in himself: the strangeness of what is destined to remain unknown to him about the fate of his identifications. The truth of the statement depends on the modalities through which the text succeeds in convincing ... in the assertion of the author's convictions.

The infantile belief, held by both writer and reader, in the possibility of rendering truly readable the way someone sees himself is an illusion that creates the truth for both parties, in an intimate register related neither to real events nor to the identificatory power of characters in a fictional text. Rather, what is offered here is the possibility of imagining how one is *likely* to be seen in the other's eyes, a lure as much for oneself as for the other—for both writer and reader—a shared illusion despite separate psychic spaces, created through sharing the words of the writing declared by oneself to be self-writing.

* * *

In other words, this approach to self-writing opposes giving the self a central role. "Self" refers to the experience of oneself described in the writing, not to a narcissistic agency,[9] nor an identity guaranteed by the supposedly unifying power of a statement or a narrative.[10]

In fact, the use of the digression just described is more and more *common*, aside from the question of self in writing, to (re)define the analytic process and its therapeutic function. But achieving therapeutic effects for the patient does not depend any more on the construction of a narrative than it does on the renewed effectiveness of a statement; it depends on the emergence of discourse related to the investigation of his psychic functioning, in the transferential address.

The autobiographical aim of discourse in analysis could be considered a belief of the patient, destined to be abandoned, even if with some patients—no doubt the most difficult—the belief persists. In the borderline sphere, the aim is to become able to let go of the belief of being oneself, and face the threat—only the threat—of disappearing. Here, we should mention the well-known opposition between narration and discourse, as it was introduced by Émile Benveniste, and developed by Gérard Genette: the narration (presented in the imperfect tense and in the third person) of a series of events, and discourse (in the present tense) as a statement addressed by an *I* to a *you*, producing an interlocution.[11] Indeed, autobiographical expression delivers a discourse presented as narration, in all its forms, from actual autobiography to Freudian self-presentation, and including autobiographical attempts—constituting a compulsion or a constraint—which bias the analytic discourse in the session.

No doubt the experience of oneself described in writing could allude to the Winnicottian self, in a perspective resembling the "primary ego-feeling" invoked by Freud in reference to a delimitation which ensures a clearly demarcated ego.[12] Thus, we can submit the idea that the writing presents an *impression* of feeling real (alive): "I am."[13] These well-known formulations, which constitute the foundations of Winnicott's view of the self, have given rise to brilliant commentary by J.-B. Pontalis who, along with André Green, introduced Winnicott's work in France. By considering the self, in a Winnicottian perspective, as the agency which makes psychic functioning "a *living* reality," Pontalis seemed to have outlined a metapsychological approach to the self as a "guardian of the feeling of existing"[14]—in 1975!

More fundamentally, halfway between ordinary language and philosophical language—specifically in phenomenology, the "self" in self-writing refers to the reflexivity of "oneself," to the self-reflexive division of internal experience: to the two-in-one of internal alterity, as it is made manifest in writing. It is also the self-reflexivity discussed by linguists, whether as a general property of language—the self-representation at the heart of all representation[15]—or, more specifically, of the "relation to the self, established in the act of designating oneself."[16]

The term "self-writing" is used to name the presentation, in writing, of a personal scene; or, more exactly, the transposition of the feeling of aliveness in one's experiencing of oneself, in the Winnicottian sense. By its very nature, this staging presumes a point of view, an awareness (recognition) that this scene is created *as if from the inside*—a perspective that can be connected to a singular *I*, who can think through, in the process of writing, his relation to himself and to the *I* of the other.[17] Defined in this manner, the term does not interfere with the identificatory postulate of a self, or with the fact that it replaces the ego of Freud's second topography, driving the division of the subject into the background.

After blinding himself irrevocably, Oedipus addressed himself to himself. Laurence Kahn has commented brilliantly on this tragic address, which transforms Oedipus into someone else: "An address to oneself ... and an address to the other in oneself."[18] Self-writing intends to write this address, openly ignoring the impossibility of such an act. In other words, self-writing promises to *feel* the truth of the fact that the author (himself) embodies the experience of addressing oneself, that is, producing the illusory writing of a personal assertion of identity. This illusion is necessary to everyone, to some degree, even outside the sphere of writing, to help the subject endure internal division, that is, experience his internal space as a conflictual relation between the single and the multiple, and as the site of a two-in-one duplexity possibly risking to turn into a duel.

The "self" in self-writing does not presuppose the theoretical postulate of an as-signable and verifiable identity, one-and-indivisible, possibly the object of despotic self-narration. Self-writing limits itself to presenting personal modes of belief—always costly and necessary to some extent, depending on the subjective particu-larities of the author—in this identity and in its verifiability by the other, *but in the intimacy of one's own psychic functioning*.[19] Through these personal modalities, self-writing exerts the necessary lure, placing faith—but not excessive faith—in an identificatory relation between the self and oneself, between the self and self-(re) presentation, between the identificatory figures of the others in oneself, and the narcissistic dimensions of one's relation to others.

* * *

This is why I consider it essential not to be content with this pseudo-evidence, so easily accepted, and perhaps even more so by psychoanalysts: that all writ-ing is self-writing, since to write always amounts to putting oneself in writing. Thus, even though Pontalis distinguishes between "writing about oneself" and "writing the self"[20] with the acuity and force of conviction he draws from his ex-perience with the different modalities of his own writing, he ultimately reduces autobiography to a "particular form of fiction."[21] In my view, this distinction could readily be applied to two positions; the first is predominant in self-writing, the second in the writing of fiction: to take hold of writing/to be gripped by writing.

My intention when I borrowed Foucault's term "self-writing"[22] as early as 1995—despite its drawbacks and despite my recourse to the plural—was to move away from an approach connected with established literary genres; and, above all, to describe a mode of literary investigation, conducted in a very specific trans-ferential sphere shared with the reader. The undertaking is literary, of course, but also psychoanalytical in several ways. Psychoanalysis is likely to offer a specific approach to self-writing, because this writing is involved in the Freudian model of self-presentation, and in the original utilisation of writing in the first person, in Freud's creative process. Thus, each psychoanalyst inherits a personal relationship with writing, whether or not he writes—that is, he inherits a specific experience of the intimacy of writing and of speech in the analytic situation.

The important thing is the status conferred on this intimacy; Pontalis sees it as a "kinship" with the power of transforming loss into absence.[23] Are psychoanalysts condemned to identify or counter-identify with Freud's envy of writers? In that case, they would have to choose between two options in their endeavour to give psychoanalysis a new beginning by finding a personal way of becoming analysts,[24] knowing that Freud's transference on writing enabled him to invent both psychoa-nalysis and a personal way of writing *I*.

The first option would be to relinquish the search for a personal way of writing *I*, by giving up writing, or by writing *like*—Freud, but also Lacan, Winnicott, etc., based on a logic of belonging, an identificatory rather than identifying logic—, while tending to reduce writing to a communications tool (of a scientific nature). The second option could be formulated as follows: *become* a writer of fiction, based on the very dubious certainty that only fiction can transmit to some extent the unprecedented experience of speech in the analytic setting. Indeed, this option is coherent with bringing into question the specificity of self-writing, considered an impoverished variant of fiction. Such a variant is much less likely than outright fiction to allow the author to *write about himself as he is*.

The present work rejects this alternative and supports the legitimacy and dignity of another mode of writing, chosen, in fact, by a number of analysts who generally lay no explicit claim to it. This mode of writing is characterised by the search for a personal manner of writing *I*, based on experiencing, in the analytic setting, a presence, in the act of listening, which is able to embody absence in the lack of response to the transferential demand, while holding out the possibility of an addressed discourse.

Here, the aim of writing is to take the risk—more or less visibly—of self-presentation, through any literary means, and whether or not there is a clinical presentation. This is a high expectation, because the self-presentation is put forth in the form of writing rooted in a singular experience without equivalent: to render present the absence of the object of transference. At the same time, the analyst inherits from Freud his transference on writing: a transference originating in the absence of the analyst and in his creative absence to himself, described by Freud in his self-presentation.

In its discussion of subjects ranging from self-writing to the psychoanalyst's writing, *The Loss of Self* intends to shed light on borderline psychopathology. An internal scene, to be imagined *as if one could see it* in the words put forth to be heard: this is what is missing in borderline psychopathology. What is lacking is a suitable place in which to feel oneself exist, a place whose borders are sufficiently well-defined and open to authorise free internal circulation. Such a place is presumed to engage in lively interaction with the "resting-place" Winnicott theorised so admirably. This area of experiencing, free of all relational obligations, connected in the *infans* with the solitary experience of having to exist, will make it possible for an entire lifetime to be alone in the presence of the other: the others in oneself, the other and his others.

Testimony to one's place—the place of being, the place where one can be—in writing: self-writing defined in this manner reveals the intention to succeed precisely where borderline existence *proclaims itself*, as always, already condemned to fail. This writing makes it possible to locate that which overcomes the impediment to being, characteristically seen in borderline patients. Indeed, I would say that this condition condemns the subject to survive his own survival, rejecting the desire to become the subject of his desire to live; as if the desire to live exposes him to the risk of having to lose his life in order not to disappear, unless he can inscribe absence in his life for good.

* * *

The reader is asked to consider this *addendum* an expression of the author's transference on psychoanalysis, that is, of his personal manner of submitting psychoanalysis to psychoanalytic questioning. This questioning lies at the heart of the analyst's transferential offer of transference, as he is spontaneously impelled to make it in the session.

Notes

1 Regardless of literary genres: autobiography, diary, autofiction, essay …
2 First formulated as such in 1999: Chiantaretto, J.-F., "L'écriture de soi à la puberté: une approche théorico-clinique. À propos des *Journaux* d'Anne Frank," *Adolescence*, 17 (1), 1999: 171–191.
3 Of these writers, Imre Kertész is and will no doubt remain an emblematic figure for me.
4 Whether the object of interpretation is the author himself—as in psychobiography and its variants—or the text with its non-explicit contents, including unconscious contents, here and there the text is reduced to what interpretation reveals: to the power the latter grants itself. From our point of view, it is not the reader-analyst who interprets the text, but the text who interprets the analyst: makes his transference interpretable, and responds to his expectation of being conceived of in the words of the other.
5 This thinking is produced by the writing itself—the writer's skill and depth of knowledge aside—in a creative compromise with repression.
6 Freud's presentation of the conception of psychoanalysis enacts the self-conception of phantasy inherent to autobiographical writing: to narrate one's conception, to conceive of oneself.
7 This reading mode, presented in 1995 in *De l'acte autobiographique*, relies on a psychoanalytic perspective and on the Freudian model of self-presentation to expand on Philippe Lejeune's idea: a reading pact proposed by the text and by its editorial presentation—a reading mode making it possible to differentiate autobiographical texts from fictional texts. See Lejeune, P., *Le Pacte autobiographique*, Seuil, 1975.
8 These forms were introduced by Serge Doubrovsky, the inventor of autofiction. See Doubrovsky, S., *Fils*, Paris: Galilée, 1977.
9 A concept best represented by Kohut, H., *Le Soi*, PUF, 1974.
10 See Schafer, R., *L'Attitude analytique*, PUF, 1988; Paul Ricoeur, *Soi-même comme un autre*, Seuil, 1990. These two authors are at the origin of the digression that led Peter Fonagy to the idea of self-narration as the aim of analytic treatment, as a clarification of a latent or potential story (see Kahn, L, *Faire parler le destin*, Klincksieck, 2005; *Psychanalysis, Apathy, and the Postmodern Patient*, Routledge, 2018.
11 See the commentary in Arrivé, M. "Histoire, discours: retour sur quelques difficultés de lecture," *Lynx*, 9, 1997: 159–168.
12 Freud, S., *Civilization and Its Discontents*, S.E. 21, Hogarth.
13 Winnicott, D., "*Sum*, I am", in *The Collected Works of D. W. Winnicott*, Vol. 8, Oxford University Press, 2016 [1968].
14 Pontalis, J.-B., "The Birth and Recognition of the 'Self,'" in *Between the Dream and Psychic Pain*, International Universities Press, 1981 [1975].
15 Recanati, F., *La Transparence et l'énonciation*, Seuil, 1979. The book looks at all the questions raised by philosophers of language and by linguists concerning the relation between the representation of the "psychical act" and its reflexivity.
16 Descombes, V., *Le Complément du sujet*, Gallimard, 2004, p. 20. The author points out the central place this question holds in debates about subject philosophy, which came under criticism by Wittgenstein.
17 Aulagnier, P., *The Violence of Interpretation*, Sheridan, A. (Trans.), Routledge, 2001.

18 Kahn, L., *Faire parler le destin*, Klincksieck, 2005.
19 This book could also be considered a protest against the present-day tendency—including on the part of certain psychoanalysts—to reduce the intimate not only to a personal trait, but to characteristics associated with an individual in full possession of the *space* of his interiority. This, despite the fact that, by its very nature, the intimate eludes the individual subject, given its hybrid composition: both phantasmatic and relational. The intimate: that which, in oneself, enlivens the relation to the other, and is enlivened by this relation.
20 Pontalis, J.-B., "Écrire pour soi ? Rêver pour qui?," in Gantheret, F. and Pontalis, J.-B. (eds.), *Parler avec l'étranger*, Gallimard, 2003.
21 Pontalis, J.-B., *La Force d'attraction*, Seuil, 1990, p. 108.
22 Foucault, M., "L'écriture de soi," *Corps écrit*, 5, 1983. Foucault's language is loaded with the controversial connotations of his later work: his battle against the Christian literature of confession—the obligation to speak of oneself. In his discussion of self-care, he opposes this literature to Ancient Greek Philosophy, free of the idea of the truth as an obligation (Foucault, M., *Dire vrai sur soi-même*, Vrin, 2017).
23 Pontalis, J.-B., *La Force d'attraction*, Seuil, 1990, p. 99.
24 In the sense that it will always be necessary, with every patient, to *become* a psychoanalyst, rather than *be* one.

Index

absence xiii, xiv, xv, xvii, xviii, xix, xx,
4–6, 8, 13, 17, 21, 26, 27, 34, 41, 45, 46,
55, 57, 58, 66, 67, 78, 82, 86, 88, 95, 96,
100, 101, 103, 104, 113, 115, 118, 119;
-capacity for absence xiv
action xiii, xiv, xix, 3, 10, 16, 29, 40, 54,
69, 76, 81, 110; -countertransferential
36, 37; -suicidal xviii; -therapeutic 30
affect xiv, xv, 7, 20, 26, 30, 37, 38, 42, 48,
54, 61; -countertransferential xv, 17,
41, 42
aftermath 9, 15, 25, 27, 30, 37, 44, 48,
56, 57, 63, 69, 74, 77, 81, 85, 97, 100,
112, 114
aliveness 101, 117
alteration 115
alterity xiii, xv, xvi, xx, 16, 20, 36, 41, 45,
63, 71, 100, 104, 115, 117
analysable: -unanalysable 18, 46, 58, 91
analysis xv, xvi, xix, 3, 5, 10, 13, 15, 17,
26–29, 31, 32, 34–39, 41, 43–45, 47, 48,
54–60, 72, 86, 91–94, 100, 104, 105, 110–
112, 115, 116; -mutual xx, 28, 35, 36, 111
analytic process xv, 5, 6, 16, 17, 43,
106, 116
anticipation xv
anxiety xv, xvi, xix, 6, 53, 92, 106
Anzieu, D. 6, 13–16, 22, 27
Appelfeld, A. 61, 62
Arendt, H. 108
Arrivé, M. 120
Aulagnier, P. xxi, 19, 20, 22, 23, 36, 95–97,
99, 103, 107, 108, 120
authentic xi; -authenticity 113
autobiography xi, xiii, 4, 15, 71, 117, 118,
120; -autobiographical xi, 10, 14, 15,
22, 61, 80, 81, 103–105, 108, 114, 116,
117, 120
autoeroticism 19, 54, 87
avoidance 6, 7

Baldacci, J.-L. 45, 49
beginning(s) 9, 13–15, 17, 18, 21, 22,
25–27, 29, 40, 46, 48, 51, 53, 58, 111;
-new beginning(s) xii, 21, 26, 29, 40,
46, 48, 51, 53, 58, 111
belief 27, 40, 42, 100
beyond survival 61, 62
body 14, 37, 54–56, 61, 81, 82, 84, 85, 87,
107, 112
borderline xviii, xx, 23, 40, 42, 45, 57, 64,
88, 89, 100, 101, 106; -existence xii, 87,
88, 106, 107, 119; -functioning xvii, 43,
50, 57, 58, 101; -patient xiii, xviii, xix,
xx, 37, 40, 41, 44, 45, 53, 89–91, 106,
119; -practice 25; -(psycho)pathologies
xi, xii, xv, xvi, 40, 52, 88, 92, 94, 97,
101, 105, 113, 119; -sphere xiv, xviii,
xix, xx, 25, 40–42, 45, 54, 57, 88, 96,
106, 116; -state xii, 25, 56, 88; -structure
xvi, 92; -subject xvi, xviii, 96, 106;
-transference 40, 41, 91

construction xii, 9, 10, 15, 21, 25, 30,
33, 51, 54, 63, 68, 71, 81, 85, 94, 96,
97, 103, 116; -deconstruction 115;
-reconstruction 9, 11, 30, 81, 84
constraint xviii, 17, 19, 104, 117
countertransference 17, 30, 35–37, 42–44,
49, 57, 89, 104, 110
countertransferential 37, 41, 93; -actions
36, 37; -affects xv, 17, 41, 42; -offer
42, 99

demand 40, 42, 47, 60, 64, 95, 99, 101,
105, 106, 119
denial xvi, 74, 83–85, 90, 94, 100, 103,
104, 106, 115
depression xxi, 43, 49, 54, 96, 101, 107,
108, 110; -depressive capacity xiii
depressivity xiii

Descombes, V. 120
desire xix, 5, 9, 15, 19–21, 31, 53, 58, 59,
    75, 81, 95, 102, 107, 110, 111, 119;
    -analyst's desire 44, 45
detachability xviii, 60
detachment xii, xviii, 91
De Toledo, C. 108
disavowal 6, 67, 85, 90, 103, 115
disillusionment 67
Doubrovsky, S. 120

effacement xiii, xiv, xvi, xvii, xviii, xix;
    -self-effacement xiii, xvii, xviii, xix, 57,
    70, 78, 90, 91, 101, 107, 112
ego xvii, 3, 4, 34, 70, 91–94, 99, 117
ego-feeling 117
empathy 35, 36, 39; -empathic function xx
erasure 7, 41, 54, 62, 76, 78, 79, 96, 100, 105
expectation xiv, xvii, 41, 61, 78, 91, 106,
    107, 119, 120
externalisation 90
extimacy 102

Fédida, P. xv, xxi, 39, 41, 44, 49, 96, 100,
    104, 108
feeling of existing 117
Ferenczi, S. xii–xv, xviii, xx, xxi, 17, 18,
    21, 23, 25–27, 29–39, 45–53, 56–60,
    78, 82, 86, 87, 89, 91, 92, 94–96, 106;
    -Ferenczian vii, xvi, 19, 26, 28, 29, 40,
    43, 44, 46, 59, 60, 86, 92, 94
fictional writing 6, 112
Fonagy, P. 120
frame 16, 40, 42, 51, 70, 94, 110
Freud, S. xi, xii, xiv, xvi, xviii, xx, 3–22,
    25–36, 38, 39, 42, 45–48, 50, 52–59, 63,
    65, 75, 89, 92, 94, 96, 98, 99, 103, 105,
    107, 108, 114, 115, 118–120; -Freudian
    3, 4, 6, 7, 12, 18, 19, 21, 22, 26, 33, 35,
    50, 51, 53, 57, 59, 60, 63, 65, 92, 93, 95,
    114, 115, 117, 118, 120

Goethe, J.-W. 3–5, 7, 8, 71, 73
Granoff, W. 25
Green, A. 42, 52, 59, 108, 117
guarantor 42, 75, 110, 116
guilt xvii, 41, 49, 53, 55, 65, 66, 78, 101,
    103, 107
Guyomard, P. 44, 49

Han, B.-C. 102, 108
hatred xvi, 14, 33, 35, 47, 49, 54, 57, 60,
    63, 64, 77, 84, 85, 89, 90, 106, 110, 111;
    -self-hatred xviii, 41, 64, 69, 89, 90

Hilflosigkeit (helplessness) xvi, 53
Hoffmann, E. T. A. 8
Holocaust xiii, 61, 63, 64, 69, 71–75, 78,
    83, 84, 100, 114

identification xv, 3, 5, 7, 14–16, 28, 33,
    37, 40, 44, 45, 58–60, 82, 90, 115, 116;
    -counter-identification 5, 15, 44, 45, 59
identificatory figure xx, 118
identity 3, 6, 7, 14, 26, 58, 65, 69–71, 76,
    83, 85, 103, 115–118
illusion 5, 17, 113, 115–117
incestuality xv, 94; -incestual xx, 56, 58,
    82, 94
incorporation xii, xvi, xviii, 15, 28, 56, 82,
    90, 94, 101, 106, 108
indivisible 3, 102, 103, 115, 118
infans xii, xvi, 19, 20, 34, 36, 40, 87, 90,
    91, 93–97, 107, 119
inner experience 63, 105
inner space 17
interlocution 11, 16, 17, 37, 47, 117;
    -internal 36, 37, 41, 42, 45, 63, 91, 103
internal: -dialogue xi, xii, xiv, xv, xvi, xvii,
    xviii, xix, xx, xxi, 18, 21, 37, 41, 47, 58,
    59, 68, 69, 71; -scene xx, 47, 61, 115,
    119; -space xx, 8, 37, 60, 117
interpretation xiv, xv, 7, 16, 20, 22, 23, 30,
    31, 35–37, 40–42, 54, 60, 78, 91, 96,
    105, 107, 114, 120

Kertész, I. xi, xiii, 61–73, 120
Khan, L. 73

Lacan, J. 6, 14–16, 25, 44, 45, 49,
    102, 118
Laplanche, J. xvi, 9, 22, 92
Levi, P. xi, 61, 62, 67, 70, 74–79
libidinal xviii, 55, 87, 101; –investment xiv,
    53, 55, 56, 70, 110; -space 99
loss viii, xii, xiii, xiv, xv, xvii, xix, 4–6, 20,
    21, 55, 57, 65, 89, 93, 103, 107, 110,
    111, 118
loss of self xii, xiii, 90, 113, 114, 119
Lugrin, Y. 27

melancholia xvi, xviii, 34, 60, 91, 101
melancholic xiii, 54, 56, 57, 84, 91, 104;
    -aspect xii, xvi, xviii, 57; -position 56;
    -threat 6, 101
melancholiform xii, 101, 107
melancholised 57
Miller, A. 80–86
Miller, M. 62, 80–86

narcissistic xii, 4, 19, 40, 47, 48, 53–55, 63, 75, 87, 89, 90, 94, 95, 99, 112, 113, 118; -ego 34, 91; -foundations 53, 87; -identification 37, 90; -injury xvi; -investment xii, xviii, 20, 52, 53, 55, 87, 90; -pleasure 102; -self-splitting xvii
narration 56, 61, 71, 104, 117, 118
narrative 15, 16, 66, 71, 85, 104, 116
narrator 14, 68, 70, 103, 115
Nebenmensch 34
negativity 31, 64, 71
new start xii, 17, 18, 25, 27, 29, 30, 45, 92

objectivation 90
obsession 14, 29; -obsessional 101
Œdipal xv, 7, 20, 48, 95
one for two xix
origin(s) vii, 3, 4, 6, 9–14, 18, 20, 21, 25, 26, 29, 33, 34, 45, 57, 59, 78, 108, 111, 115, 120
original xii, 9–11, 13, 17–20, 25, 26, 28, 45, 46, 48, 58, 59, 65, 78, 81, 91, 93, 114, 115, 118
originary vii, xii, xiv, 9–14, 17, 19, 20, 25, 58, 65, 78, 85, 89, 115
otherness xii

Pachet, P. xiii, xxi
paradox 27, 33, 102, 115
paradoxical 5, 19, 28, 41, 55, 57, 66, 69, 89, 90, 101, 115
Perrier, F. xvi, xxi, 96
perverse 19, 23
phantasy 4, 9–12, 15, 18, 20–22, 103–105, 110, 115, 120; -phantasmatic 9, 12, 19, 29, 48, 58, 81, 110, 115, 121
Pingeot, M. 101, 108
Pontalis, J.-B. xxi, 8, 9, 13–15, 22, 117, 118, 120, 121
potential writing xvii, 17
presence xiv, xv, xvi, xx, 27, 28, 35, 36, 40–42, 55, 58, 59, 64, 68, 71, 75, 76, 87–91, 94–96, 99, 100, 103, 105–107, 113, 119
primal scene 4, 6, 9, 11, 12, 18–20, 26, 45
psychoanalytic cure 4
psychosis 93, 105
psychotherapy 39, 109, 111, 112
psychotic 60, 88, 92, 105

Racamier, P.-C. 94, 96
Recanati, F. 108, 120
reciprocity xiv, xv
regression 28, 43, 49

relational xii, xx, 60, 75, 78, 96, 119; -incapacity 78
resistance xvii, xx, 4, 8, 17, 27, 31, 35, 44, 45, 58, 75, 92, 99–101, 105, 106, 111, 114
Ricoeur, P. 120
Rolland, J.-C. xxi
Rosenberg, B. xviii, xxi, 60
Royer, C. 72, 73

Schafer, R. 120
Searles, H. 53, 60, 88
self-writing 62, 88
session xii–xx, 3, 6, 8, 17, 26, 36, 37, 39, 42, 43, 48, 54–56, 58, 82, 100, 101, 104, 109, 112, 114, 117, 120
Severn, E. 37
shared sphere xviii
site of the stranger xv, xvi, xxi, 45, 49
splitting xvii, 56, 83, 85; -narcissistic self-splitting xvi, xvii
Starobinski, J. 103, 108
strangeness 45, 46, 78, 94
soul murder xvii, 45, 46, 78, 94
subject xi, xii, xiii, xvi, xviii, 6, 8–11, 16, 18–22, 27, 28, 33, 45, 47, 52, 54, 63, 64, 66, 75, 77–79, 81, 82, 87–89, 94–96, 98–101, 103–107, 115, 117, 119–121
subjectivity 75, 100
subjectless 54
subject supposed to know 6
superego 4, 5, 28, 98, 99
supervision xiv, xvii, xviii, 35–37, 82
survival xi, xiv, xvi, xx, 36, 61–63, 66, 68, 69, 71, 74, 78, 81, 85, 88–90, 95, 106, 114, 119
symbolic community 38
symbolisation xv, 57

tact 30, 35, 53; -tactful 51
testimony 4, 10, 12, 68, 72, 74, 81, 85, 100, 103, 115, 119
the being xvii, xx, 17, 20, 87; -component of xx; -division of xvii
thinking process xi, xiv, xvii, xix, 16, 17, 20, 29, 38, 45, 84, 92, 95, 106
third 6, 20, 29, 31, 41, 58, 59, 68, 75, 77, 82, 110, 117; -element 4; -function xx
thirdness xiv, xviii, xix, xx, 16, 29, 37, 45, 59, 81, 85; -space of xviii, 37
transcription xi, xvii
transference xii–xx, 3, 5–7, 10, 11, 16–18, 25, 27–31, 33, 35–46, 48, 49, 55, 57, 58,

85, 90–92, 101, 104–106, 110, 112, 114, 115, 118–120; -analyst's xix, 5, 18, 21, 42, 43, 59, 109; -on (psycho)analysis 33, 45
transferential xv, xvi, xvii, xix, 5, 10, 17, 25–27, 30–32, 34, 36, 37, 40, 41, 44, 46–48, 54, 56–59, 91, 93, 94, 109, 110, 114, 116; -demand 99, 105, 106, 119; -depression 43; -induction xiv; -object xiii, 42; -offer 11, 28, 99, 101, 120; -(role) attribution xiv, xvii, 10, 57; -writing 109
transgression 18, 19, 21–23, 105
transparency 98, 100–105, 107, 108
trauma 7, 28, 30, 33, 35, 64, 75, 78, 93
traumatic xiii, 8, 28, 30, 34, 36, 67, 69, 70, 74, 75, 78, 94

unthinkable xiv, 6, 7, 40, 48, 92, 93, 95, 106, 114
unwelcome xxi, 23, 28, 35, 40, 46, 50, 55–59, 96, 106, 110

Widlöcher, D. 37, 39
Winnicott, D. H. xxi, 6, 25, 36, 37, 39, 42–44, 48, 49, 52, 53, 57, 59, 60, 78, 87, 89, 92–96, 117–120; -Winnicottian xiv, 19, 42, 52, 91, 95, 105, 111, 117
witness xi, xiii, xiv, 3, 4, 9, 11, 13, 15, 17, 21, 22, 30, 36, 41, 45, 47, 56, 58, 61, 63, 64, 68, 71, 74, 75, 77, 80–82, 85, 103, 106, 107, 110, 113, 115, 116
work of culture 99
work of melancholia xviii, 60, 101
work of mourning 81
writing as thinking process xi, xvii, xix